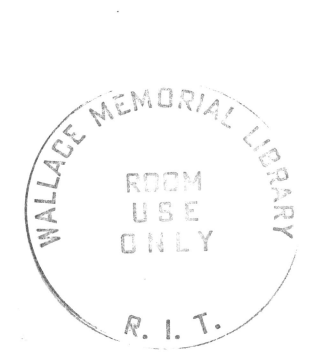

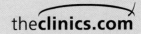

RADIOLOGIC
CLINICS
OF NORTH AMERICA

Update on PET/CT Imaging

July 2007 • Volume 45 • Number 4

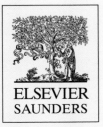

ELSEVIER
SAUNDERS

An imprint of Elsevier, Inc
PHILADELPHIA LONDON TORONTO MONTREAL SYDNEY TOKYO

W.B. SAUNDERS COMPANY
A Division of Elsevier Inc.

1600 John F. Kennedy Boulevard • Suite 1800 • Philadelphia, Pennsylvania 19103-2899

http://www.theclinics.com

RADIOLOGIC CLINICS OF NORTH AMERICA Volume 45, Number 4
July 2007 ISSN 0033-8389, ISBN-13: 978-1-4160-5120-6; ISBN-10: 1-4160-5120-1

Editor: Barton Dudlick

Reprints: For copies of 100 or more, of articles in this publication, please contact the Commercial Reprints Department, Elsevier Inc., 360 Park Avenue South, New York, New York 10010-1710. Tel.: (+1) 212-633-3813; Fax: (+1) 212-462-1935; E-mail: reprints@elsevier.com.

The ideas and opinions expressed in *Radiologic Clinics of North America* do not necessarily reflect those of the Publisher does not assume any responsibility for any injury and/or damage to persons or property arising out of or related to any use of the material contained in this periodical. The reader is advised to check the appropriate medical literature and the product information currently provided by the manufacturer of each drug to be administered to verify the dosage, the method and duration of administration, or contraindications, It is the responsibility of the treating physician or other health care professional, relying on independent experience and knowledge of the patient, to determine drug dosages and the best treatment for the patient. Mention of any product in this issue should not be construed as endorsement by the contributiors, editors, or the Publisher of the productor manufacturers' claims.

Radiologic Clinics of North America (ISSN 0033-8389) is published bimonthly in January, March, May, July, September, and November by Elsevier Inc., 360 Park Avenue South, New York, NY 10010-1710. Business and editorial offices: 1600 John F. Kenedy Boulevard, Suite 1800, Philadelphia, Pennsylvania 19103-2899. Customer Service Office: 6277 Sea Harbor Drive, Orlando, FL 32887-4800. Periodicals postage paid at New York, NY, and additional mailing offices. Subscription prices are USD 259 per year for US individuals, USD 385 per year for US institutions, USD 127 per year for US students and residents, USD 303 per year for Canadian individuals, USD 473 per year of Canadian institutions, USD 352 per year for international individuals, USD 473 per year for international institutions, and USD 171 per year for Canadian and foreign students/residents. To receive student and resident rate, orders must be accompanied by name of affiliated institution, date of term, and the signature of program/residency coordinatior on institution letterhead. Orders will be billed at individual rate until proof of status is received. Foreign air speed delivery is included in all Clinics subscriptionprices. All prices are subject to change without notice. **POSTMASTER:** Send address changes to *Radiologic Clinics of North America*, Elsevier Periodicals Customer Service, 6277 Sea Harbor Drive, Orlando, FL 32887-4800. **Customer Service: 1-800-654-2452 (US). From outside of the US, call (+1) 407-345-4000.**

Radiologic Clinics of North America also published in Greek Paschalidis Medical Publications, Athens, Greece.

Radiologic Clinics of North America is covered in *Index Medicus, EMBASE/Excerpta Medica, Current Contents/Life Sciences, Current Contents/Clinical Medicine, RSNA Index to Imaging Literature, BIOSIS, Science Citation Index,* and *ISI/BIOMED.*

Printed in the United States of America.

UPDATE ON PET/CT IMAGING

CONTRIBUTORS

LEE P. ADLER, MD
Adler Institute for Advanced Imaging, Jenkintown, Pennsylvania

ABASS ALAVI, MD
Professor and Chief, Division of Nuclear Medicine, Department of Radiology, University of Pennsylvania Medical Center, Philadelphia, Pennsylvania

GERALD ANTOCH, MD
Department of Diagnostic and Interventional, Radiology, University of Duisburg, Essen, Germany

NORBERT AVRIL, MD
Associate Professor, Department of Nuclear Medicine, Barts and the London School of Medicine, Queen Mary, University of London, West Smithfield, London, United Kingdom

RACHEL BAR-SHALOM, MD
Director, Division of Positron Emission Tomography, Department of Nuclear Medicine, Rambam Health Care Campus; and B. Rapaport School of Medicine, Israel Institute of Technology-Technion, Haifa, Israel

THOMAS BEYER, PhD
Department of Nuclear Medicine, University of Duisburg, Essen, Germany

ANDREAS BOCKISCH, MD, PhD
Department of Nuclear Medicine, University of Duisburg, Essen, Germany

CHRISTOPHE DOOMS, MD
Respiratory Oncology Unit (Pulmonology), Leuven Lung Cancer Group, University Hospital Gasthuisberg, Catholic University, Leuven, Belgium

WILLIAM B. EUBANK, MD
Associate Professor, Department of Radiology, Puget Sound Veterans Administration Health Care System, Seattle, Washington

EINAT EVEN-SAPIR, MD, PhD
Department of Nuclear Medicine, Tel-Aviv Sourasky Medical Center, Sackler Faculty of Medicine, Tel-Aviv University, Tel-Aviv, Israel

LUTZ S. FREUDENBERG, MD, MA, MBA
Department of Nuclear Medicine, University of Duisburg, Essen, Germany

YAIR HERISHANU, MD
Department of Hematology, Tel-Aviv Sourasky Medical Center, Sackler Faculty of Medicine, Tel-Aviv University, Tel-Aviv, Israel

RODNEY J. HICKS, MD, FRACP
Professor, Centre for Molecular Imaging, Peter MacCallum Cancer Centre, East Melbourne, Victoria, Australia

HEDVA LERMAN, MD
Department of Nuclear Medicine, Tel-Aviv Sourasky Medical Center, Sackler Faculty of Medicine, Tel-Aviv University, Tel-Aviv, Israel

TORSTEN LIERSCH, MD
Department of General Surgery, University of Göttingen, Göttingen, Germany

GENADY LIEVSHITZ, MD
Department of Nuclear Medicine, Tel-Aviv Sourasky Medical Center, Sackler Faculty of Medicine, Tel-Aviv University, Tel-Aviv, Israel

HOMER A. MACAPINLAC, MD
Chairman Ad Interim and Associate Professor, University of Texas, M.D. Anderson Cancer Center, Houston, Texas

MICHAEL P. MAC MANUS, MD, MRCP, FRCR, FFRRCSI, FRANZCR
Associate Professor, Department of Radiation Oncology, Peter MacCallum Cancer Centre, East Melbourne, Victoria, Australia

JOHANNES MELLER, MD
Adjunct Professor and Director, Department of Nuclear Medicine, University of Göttingen, Göttingen, Germany

UR METSER, MD
Department of Nuclear Medicine, Tel-Aviv Sourasky Medical Center, Sackler Faculty of Medicine, Tel-Aviv University, Tel-Aviv, Israel

CHAVA PERRY, MD
Department of Hematology, Tel-Aviv Sourasky
Medical Center, Sackler Faculty
of Medicine, Tel-Aviv University, Tel-Aviv, Israel

DONALD A. PODOLOFF, MD
Head and Professor, Division of Diagnostic
Imaging, University of Texas, M.D. Anderson
Cancer Center, Houston, Texas

SANDRA J. ROSENBAUM, MD
Department of Nuclear Medicine, University
of Duisburg, Essen, Germany

CARSTEN OLIVER SAHLMANN, MD
Department of Nuclear Medicine, University
of Göttingen, Göttingen, Germany

HOLGER SCHIRRMEISTER, MD
Consultant of Nuclear Medicine, Clinic of Nuclear
Medicine, University of Kiel, Kiel, Germany

SIGRID STROOBANTS, MD, PhD
PET Center (Nuclear Medicine), University
Hospital Gasthuisberg, Catholic University, Leuven,
Belgium

PETER HAO TANG, BA
Research Coordinator, Division of Nuclear
Medicine, Department of Radiology, Hospital of

the University of Pennsylvania, Philadelphia,
Pennsylvania

JOHAN VANSTEENKISTE, MD, PhD
Respiratory Oncology Unit (Pulmonology), Leuven
Lung Cancer Group, University Hospital
Gasthuisberg, Catholic University, Leuven, Belgium

MARTIN A. WALTER, MD
Institute of Nuclear Medicine, University Hospital
Basel, Basel, Switzerland

JOKKE WYNANTS, MD
Respiratory Oncology Unit (Pulmonology),
Leuven Lung Cancer Group, University Hospital
Gasthuisberg, Catholic University, Leuven,
Belgium

HUA YANG, MD
Division of Nuclear Medicine, Department
of Radiology, University of Pennsylvania School
of Medicine, Hospital of the University of
Pennsylvania, Philadelphia, Pennsylvania

HONGMING ZHUANG, MD, PhD
Chief, Division of Nuclear Medicine, The Children's
Hospital of Philadelphia; and Assistant Professor,
Department of Radiology, University of
Pennsylvania School of Medicine, Philadelphia,
Pennsylvania

UPDATE ON PET/CT IMAGING

Volume 45 · Number 4 · July 2007

Contents

clinically significant interpretation that has an impact on patient management and potentially on outcome.

Donald A. Podoloff and Homer A. Macapinlac

Within recent years, F-18 fluorodeoxyglucose (FDG) PET has become the most important nuclear medicine and radiology imaging modality in the management of lymphoma. FDG-PET detects more disease sites and involved organs than conventional staging procedures, including CT, and has a large influence on staging. FDG-PET performed during and after therapy seems to provide considerable prognostic information. The impact on patient outcome is not clear, however, because no controlled trials have yet been conducted and follow-up periods are generally short.

Einat Even-Sapir, Genady Lievshitz, Chava Perry, Yair Herishanu, Hedva Lerman, and Ur Metser

Lymphoma may originate in extranodal sites. Extranodal lymphoma may also be secondary to and accompany nodal disease. Fluorine-18 fluorodeoxyglucose (18F-FDG) imaging has an essential role in the staging of lymphoma, in monitoring the response to therapy, and in detection of recurrence. The introduction of 18F-FDG PET/CT hybrid imaging allows for accurate localization of disease and may be specifically beneficial for the detection of unexpected extranodal sites of disease or exclusion of disease in the presence of nonspecific extranodal CT findings. Accurate staging and localization often dictate the appropriate treatment strategy in patients with lymphoma. Therefore, at any stage in the course of the disease, the potential presence of extranodal disease should be considered when interpreting 18F-FDG PET/CT studies in patients with non-Hodgkin lymphoma and Hodgkin's disease.

Hongming Zhuang, Hua Yang, and Abass Alavi

The most frequent complications after arthroplasty are aseptic loosening and infection. It is often difficult to differentiate aseptic loosening from infection. The management of these two distinct clinical identities is quite different, however. Treatment of aseptic loosening usually requires one-step revision surgery, whereas treatment of infection requires antimicrobial therapy for an extended period before inserting a new prosthesis. Infection associated with arthroplasty is a serious complication and should be treated adequately before proceeding with a surgical intervention. PET with 18F-labeled fluorodeoxyglucose (FDG) has been proposed as an accurate technique for evaluating painful arthroplasty. This review addresses the applications of FDG-PET in such clinical settings. In addition, the potential of PET in the assessing the viability of bone grafts in revision arthroplasty is discussed.

Johannes Meller, Carsten Oliver Sahlmann, Torsten Liersch, Peter Hao Tang, and Abass Alavi

This article describes the impact of [18F]2-fluoro-2-deoxy-D-glucose (FDG) PET in the diagnosis of non–prosthesis-related orthopedic infections and inflammation. FDG-PET has an excellent sensitivity in the detection of osteomyelitis (OM). Early data indicate that FDG-PET may be more specific than MRI in diagnosing OM. The role of the combination of FDG and PET-CT in the diagnosis of OM is likely to be determined as this combination is used on a routine basis. Early data from studies in rheumatoid arthritis indicate that FDG-PET is highly accurate in early diagnosis and that it provides results comparable to the most advanced conventional techniques.

[^{18}F]Fluorodeoxyglucose PET in Large Vessel Vasculitis   735

Martin A. Walter

[^{18}F]fluorodeoxyglucose (FDG) PET is a noninvasive metabolic imaging modality based on the regional distribution of [18F]FDG that is highly effective in assessing the activity and extent of giant cell arteritis and Takayasu's arteritis, respectively. Metabolic imaging using [18F]FDG-PET has been shown to identify more affected vascular regions than morphologic imaging with MRI in both diseases. The visual grading of vascular [18F]FDG uptake helps to discriminate arteritis from atherosclerosis and therefore provides high specificity. High sensitivity is attained by scanning during the active inflammatory phase. Thus, [18F]FDG-PET has the potential to develop into a valuable tool in the diagnostic workup of giant cell arteritis and Takayasu's arteritis.

Index   745

RADIOLOGIC
CLINICS
OF NORTH AMERICA

Radiol Clin N Am 45 (2007) 609–625

Staging of Lung Cancer

Jokke Wynants, MD[a], Sigrid Stroobants, MD, PhD[b],
Christophe Dooms, MD[a], Johan Vansteenkiste, MD, PhD[a],*

Lung cancer is the most common cause of cancer-related death in the Western world, with approximately 1.2 million new cases per year worldwide. Imaging techniques play a vital role in the diagnosis, staging, and follow-up of patients who have lung cancer. For this purpose, PET has become an important adjunct to conventional imaging techniques such as chest radiography, CT, ultrasonography, and MR imaging [1]. The ability of PET to differentiate the metabolic properties of tissues allows more accurate assessment of undetermined lung lesions, mediastinal lymph nodes (LNs), or extrathoracic abnormalities, tumor response after induction treatment, and detection of disease recurrence [2].

The standard tracer in lung cancer PET imaging is the glucose analogue ^{18}F-fluoro-2-deoxy-D-glucose (FDG). FDG allows excellent discrimination between normal tissues and tissues with enhanced glucose metabolism, but false-positive uptake of FDG in inflammatory tissues is one of its major limitations. Therefore, tracers with an equally high sensitivity but a better specificity are the focus of ongoing research. Other tracers such as ^{11}C-methionine (a marker of protein metabolism), ^{11}C-choline (a marker of the cell membrane component phosphaditylcholine), and ^{18}F-fluoro-thymidine (a marker of cell proliferation) have been studied. The experience with these tracers is still limited. At this time they have not shown a clear advantage over FDG in clinical lung cancer imaging, and they are not discussed further in this article.

Most of the studies in lung cancer were performed with a full-ring (or "dedicated") PET camera, and they are the basis for the recommendations for the use of PET in clinical decisions. It is not clear, and is even doubtful, if the same recommendations apply to dual-head coincidence gamma camera imaging.

The staging system of lung cancer

For the past 2 decades, the international staging system for lung cancer has provided a common

This article was previously published in PET Clinics 2006;1:301–15.
 a Respiratory Oncology Unit (Pulmonology), Leuven Lung Cancer Group, University Hospital Gasthuisberg, Catholic University, Herestraat 49, B-3000, Leuven, Belgium
b PET Center (Nuclear Medicine), University Hospital Gasthuisberg, Catholic University, Herestraat 49, B-3000, Leuven, Belgium
* Corresponding author.
E-mail address: johan.vansteenkiste@uz.kuleuven.ac.be (J. Vansteenkiste).

language for communication about patients. Accurate staging is essential to make estimates of prognosis and to choose the best combination of treatment modalities such as surgery, radiotherapy, and chemotherapy in an attempt to improve survival.

The system defines the TNM category of each patient who has non–small cell lung cancer (NSCLC) (Table 1) [3]. The T factor describes the primary tumor by size and invasiveness, ranging from T1 (< 3 cm and entirely surrounded by lung tissue) to T4 (invading critical organs such as the aorta). The N factor describes the locoregional LN spread, either no metastatic nodes (N0), to intrapulmonary or hilar nodes only (N1), to ipsilateral mediastinal nodes (N2), or to contralateral mediastinal or supraclavicular nodes (N3). The M factor denotes absence (M0) or presence (M1) of distant metastasis.

A major step forward in the latest staging system has been the adoption of a unique system for N-factor staging. Previously, there were two mediastinal LN classifications, one by Naruke [4] and the other by the American Thoracic Society [5]. The map published in 1997 was recognized by the American Joint Committee on Cancer and the TNM Committee of the Union Internationale

Contre le Cancer (Fig. 1) [6]. The three groups of mediastinal LNs are indicated by a single digit: superior (1–4), aortic (5 or 6), and inferior (7–9). Hilar (10) and intrapulmonary (11–13) LNs have a double digit. This map can be used to interpret imaging studies and to guide LN sampling procedures such as endoscopic needle aspirations or mediastinoscopy [7]. The pattern of LN spread; depends, in general, on the site of the primary tumor. Right upper- and middle-lobe tumors often spread to the right hilar and right superior mediastinal nodes, right lower-lobe tumors often spread to the right hilar and inferior mediastinal stations. Left upper-lobe tumors have a predilection for left hilar, aortic, and left paratracheal nodes; left lower-lobe tumors spread to the left hilar nodes and the inferior mediastinal nodes, with a high tendency to cross the midline.

Based on their TNM denominators, patients are grouped into stages with more-or-less homogeneous prognosis. The current system distinguishes seven stages of disease, each with a different outcome (see Table 1). For therapeutic considerations, stage I and stage ,II disease are often referred to as "early stage"; for these patients the standard of care is local treatment, preferably resection followed by adjuvant chemotherapy except for stage

Table 1:	**TNM staging of lung cancer**			
Stage	**Tumor**	**Node**	**Metastasis**	**Definition**
IA	T1	N0	M0	T1 tumor: ≤3 cm, surrounded by lung or pleura; no tumor more proximal than lobe bronchus
IB	T2	N0	M0	T2 tumor: >3cm, involving main bronchus ≥2 cm distal to carina, invading pleura; atelectasis or pneumonitis extending to hilum but not entire lung
IIA	T1	N1	M0	N1: involvement of ipsilateral peribronchial or hilar nodes and intra, pulmonary nodes by direct extension
IIB	T2	N1	M0	
	T3	N0	M0	T3 tumor: invasion of chest wall, diaphragm. mediastinal pleura, pericardium, main bronchus <2 cm distal to carina; atelectasis or pneumonitis of entire lung
IIIA	T1	N2	M0	
	T2	N2	M0	
	T3	N1	M0	
	T3	N2	M0	N2: involvement ipsilateral mediastinal or subcarinal nodes
IIIB	Any T	N3	M0	N3: involvement of contralateral (lung) nodes or any supraclavicular node
IIIB	T4	Any N	M0	T4 tumor: invasion of mediastinum, heart, great vessels, trachea, esophagus, vertebral body, carina; separate tumor nodules; malignant pleural effusion
IV	Any T	Any N	M1	Distant metastasis

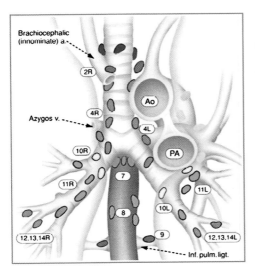

Superior Mediastinal Nodes

- ● **1** Highest Mediastinal
- ● **2** Upper Paratracheal
- ● **3** Pre-vascular and Retrotracheal
- ◑ **4** Lower Paratracheal (including Azygos Nodes)

N_2 = single digit, ipsilateral
N_3 = single digit, contralateral or supraclavicular

Aortic Nodes

- ● **5** Subaortic (A-P window)
- ● **6** Para-aortic (ascending aorta or phrenic)

Inferior Mediastinal Nodes

- ◑ **7** Subcarinal
- ● **8** Paraesophageal (below carina)
- ● **9** Pulmonary Ligament

N_1 Nodes

- ○ **10** Hilar
- ◑ **11** Interlobar
- ◑ **12** Lobar
- ◑ **13** Segmental
- ◑ **14** Subsegmental

Fig. 1. Lung cancer lymph node map according to Mountain and Dressler. Ao, aorta; L, left; N_2, single-digit, ipsilateral; N_3, single-digit, contralateral or supraclavicular; PA, pulmonary artery; R, right; 1, highest mediastinal node; 2, upper paratracheal nodes; 3, prevascular and retrotracheal nodes; 4, lower paratracheal nodes; 5, subaortic nodes (aortopulmonary window); 6, para-aortic nodes (ascending aorta or phrenic); 7, subcarinal nodes; 8, paraesophageal nodes (below carina); 9, pulmonary ligament; 10, hilar nodes; 11, interlobar nodes; 12, lobar nodes; 13, segmental nodes; 14, subsegmental nodes. (*Courtesy of* Clifton F. Mountain, MD, San Diego, CA, with permission. © Copyright 1996, Mountain and Dresler.)

IA [8], or radical radiotherapy in case of poor cardiopulmonary function. Patients who have stage III disease have locally advanced disease, either IIIA (N2: LN spread in the ipsilateral mediastinal nodes only) or IIIB (N3: LN spread in the contralateral mediastinal or supraclavicular nodes). Except for patients who have IIIB stage based on T4 malignant pleural effusion, a combination of local and systemic treatment offers the best prospects for remission, or sometimes cure. In North America, this treatment often is concurrent chemoradiotherapy [9]. Many European centers treat patients who

have stage IIIA disease with induction therapy followed by attempted complete resection [10–13]. Patients who have stage IV (advanced or metastatic) disease are no longer amenable to cure. Chemotherapy results in a moderate improvement of the median survival, subjective clinical benefit [14], or quality of life [15].

Baseline staging: T factor

In general, CT has gained a central role in lung cancer staging and now is appropriate for every treatable patient. MR imaging can be of additional benefit in some instances (eg, by showing superior sulcus extension or the relationship with the heart or large vessels) [16]. With its excellent anatomic detail, however, modern CT is the best choice to assess the T factor, that is, the relationship of the tumor to the fissures (which may determine the type of resection), to mediastinal structures, or to the pleura and chest wall. For the assessment of primary tumor extension, CT with its better spatial resolution remains the standard test. CT criteria for probable resectability in masses contiguous with the mediastinum are a contact with mediastinum of less than 3 cm, less than 90° contact with aorta, and preserved mediastinal fat layer between the mass and mediastinal structures. The reverse findings (ie, >3-cm contact with mediastinum, > 90° contact with aorta, obliteration of the fat plane between mass and mediastinal structures) are not reliable signs of either invasion or nonresectability [17–19]. Consequently, CT often does not obviate surgical exploration, because it provides reliable signs of resectability but less reliable signs of nonresectability. The same is true for chest wall invasion, with the exception of the 100% positive predictive value of bony rib destruction with or without a soft tissue mass extending into the chest wall [16,20,21].

PET by itself does not add much to the assessment of local resectability, because its inferior spatial resolution does not provide more detail of the exact tumor extent or infiltration of neighboring structures. Recently, one prospective study of 40 patients reported that PET-CT fusion images provided more precise information for the evaluation of chest wall and mediastinal infiltration in some patients because of better differentiation between tumor and peritumoral inflammation or atelectasis [22]. A review of the experience at the Leuven Lung Cancer Group (LLCG) with fusion PET-CT, in comparison with CT alone, PET alone, and side-to-side correlated PET-CT, revealed a sensitivity for fusion PET-CT of 83%, a specificity of 84%, and an accuracy of 84% [23]. These results were significantly better than for CT alone or PET alone, but there was no benefit in comparison with side-to-side correlated PET-CT.

Evaluation of pleural disease

The presence of pleural fluid in a patient who has lung cancer always should raise the possibility of pleural tumor spread, thereby changing the T factor from T1–T3 to T4 and thus changing staging to stage IIIB, no longer amenable to potentially radical therapy. Malignant pleural effusion should, however, be differentiated from nonmalignant fluid,

which can be caused by atelectasis, pneumonia, or impairment of lymphatic drainage.

In a first retrospective report on 25 patients who had NSCLC and suspected malignant pleural effusions, PET was reported to have a sensitivity of 95% (21/22 patients) [24]. Because only three patients in this series had benign pleural disease, specificity could not be judged truly. In another study with a prevalence of malignant pleural involvement of about 50%, PET correctly detected the presence of malignant pleural involvement in 16 of 18 patients and excluded malignant pleural involvement in 16 of 17 patients (sensitivity 89%, specificity 94%, accuracy 91%) [25]. In a later study of pleural effusion in 92 patients, of whom 71% were deemed indeterminate on CT, PET had a sensitivity, specificity, and accuracy of 100%, 71%, and 80%, respectively, and PET/CT had a sensitivity, specificity, and accuracy of 100%, 76%, and 84%, respectively [26]. In this particular study, specificity and positive predictive value were lower, because of the larger number of benign pleural effusions.

The outcome of these studies thus varies according to the type of patients included and the prevalence of malignancy in the total number of effusions. PET thus can be useful in evaluating pleural disease in patients who have lung cancer but nonetheless should be interpreted with caution. Small or flat pleural deposits can indeed be missed on PET, probably because of their low tumor load or partial volume effects (Fig. 2) [27]. On the other hand, false-positive findings may occur in patients who have inflammatory pleural lesions. If the pleural staging determines the chances for radical treatment, pathologic verification with cytology or thoracoscopic biopsy should be sought.

Baseline staging: N factor

The N stage describes the presence and extent of locoregional LN invasion in NSCLC, and strongly determines the prognosis and the choice of treatment when distant metastases are absent. For patients who do not have positive LNs or who have only intrapulmonary or hilar ones, direct resection remains standard therapy. In case of positive ipsilateral mediastinal LNs (N2), induction treatment followed by surgery is a choice for resectable patients; others are treated with a combination of chemotherapy and radiotherapy [10,28]. Patients who have contralateral metastatic mediastinal LNs (N3 disease) generally are not candidates for surgery but receive nonsurgical combined modality treatment.

For years CT has been the standard noninvasive staging method for the mediastinum. Enlarged LNs (ie, > 10 mm in the short axis) were considered

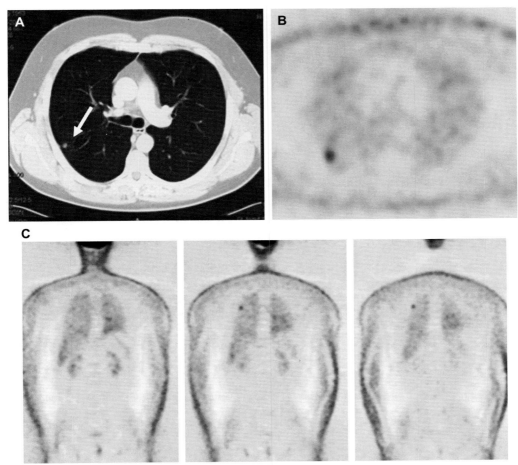

Fig. 2. (*A*) Detection of a small pulmonary nodule on a CT made for vague right-sided thoracic pain in a 41-year-old patient. (*B, C*) The lesion is FDG avid. There are no signs of lymph node or pleural disease and no explanation for thoracic pain. At thoracoscopy, diffuse superficial pleural metastases from a lung adenocarcinoma were present.

to be metastatic. Size is a relative criterion, however, because there can be infectious or inflammatory causes for LNs enlargement, and small nodes can contain metastatic deposits. The sensitivity and specificity of thoracic CT for detection of mediastinal LN spread were only 69% and 71%, respectively, in one large series [29]. In a review, the pooled sensitivity of CT was 57% (95% confidence interval [CI], 49%–66%) and the specificity was 82% (95% CI, 77%–86%) [30].

During the last years, several prospective studies yielded strong evidence that PET is significantly more accurate than thoracic CT for assessing the N factor in NSCLC. In a landmark LLCG study, PET proved significantly more accurate than CT in LN staging, and if CT and PET images were correlated, the negative predictive value of 95% proved to be slightly better than the one reported in mediastinoscopy series [31]. This superiority has been confirmed in five meta-analyses [30,32–35]. PET correctly identifies large benign nodes and also small malignant nodes because of the high contrast resolution of FDG-avid LN metastases on PET (Fig. 3). In a comparative study, the sensitivity, specificity, and accuracy of PET for detecting small (<1 cm in size) malignant LNs were 80%, 95%, and 92% respectively, and for LNs of 1 to 3 cm were 100%, 91%, and 95%, respectively [36].

The high negative predictive value is the true strength of PET. It creates the possibility of avoiding invasive staging if PET suggests the absence of LN disease. This negative predictive value is valid only when there is sufficient FDG uptake in the primary tumor and in the absence of a central tumor or important hilar LN disease that may obscure co-existing N2 disease [37]. If these rules of interpretation are observed, relevant LN disease rarely is missed. In some patients, LNs with small tumor

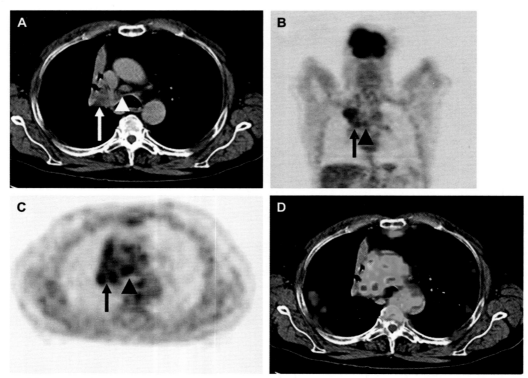

Fig. 3. (A) CT scan of a patient who has a centrally located right upper lobe tumor (*arrow*) and a small lymph node in the right paratracheal space (*arrowhead*). (B, C) FDG uptake in the tumor, hilar (*arrow*), and right mediastinal nodes (*arrowhead*). (D) Fusion images clearly suggest mediastinal lymph node spread, which was confirmed at cervical mediastinoscopy.

deposits, ranging from 1 to 7.5 mm [38], may remain undetected because of the spatial resolution of the PET camera. In these patients, minimal N2 disease may be discovered at surgical exploration, but resection in these patients is rewarding [39,40].

The positive predictive value of PET is less optimal. Therefore, in case of positive LN findings on PET, tissue confirmation is mandatory to avoid radical surgery in node-free patients based on false-positive findings (eg, caused by granulomatous or other inflammatory conditions).

The available studies indicate that visual correlation with CT images is the minimal standard to optimize PET interpretation [41–43]. Fusion PET-CT images are one step further, with the obvious advantage of decreasing the learning curve needed to optimize the visual correlation (Fig. 4). The advantages of this approach are discussed elsewhere in this issue.

Baseline staging: M factor

The observation of metastases in patients who have NSCLC implies that a patient can no longer be cured. Forty percent of the patients who have

NSCLC have distant metastases at presentation, most commonly in the adrenal glands, bones, liver, or brain [44]. The current standard noninvasive staging tests (including ultrasound, CT, MR imaging, and bone scintigraphy) are far from perfect. A systemic relapse develops in up to 20% of surgically treated patients within 3 to 24 months after complete surgical resection. The explanation of the high false-negative rate of conventional imaging probably lies in the presence of micrometastatic spread at the time of diagnosis of biologically more aggressive tumors [45].

PET offers a double additional value in the evaluation of distant metastases in patients who have potentially operable NSCLC. On the one hand, there is the detection of unexpected metastatic spread, which occurs in 5% to 29% of patients who have negative conventional imaging (Fig. 5) [46–59]. This broad range is explained by several factors. First is the variability in the extent or rigor of the pre-PET extrathoracic conventional imaging. Second, in some studies the equivocal lesions are regarded as unexpected metastases if PET confirms malignancy in these lesions [47,48], but this is not the case in most other studies. Finally, the

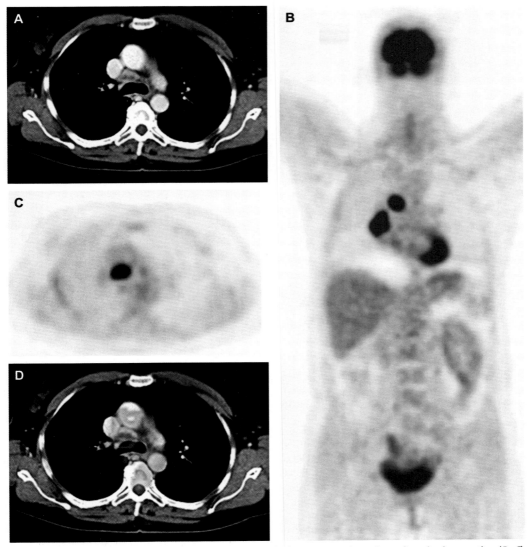

Fig. 4. (*A*) CT of a patient who has a centrally located right lung tumor (not shown) and adenopathy. (*B, C*) On PET images, adenopathy can be either right hilar, right mediastinal, or both. (*D*) Fusion images confirm that the lymph node metastasis has a right paratracheal location (4R in Fig. 1).

chance of detecting metastases on PET varies with the population in the study, being found in 7% of the patients who have pre-PET stage I disease, in 18% of patients who have stage II disease, and in up to 24% of patients who have stage III disease [53]. Focal unexpected FDG-PET uptake in sites unlikely to be metastatic for NSCLC also may reveal a second primary tumor in some patients (eg, colorectal or breast cancer) (Fig. 6).

On the other hand, lesions that are equivocal on conventional imaging can be assessed further by PET. Because of the very high sensitivity of PET in the detection of adrenal metastases, a negative PET image of an equivocal adrenal lesion on CT

usually indicates a nonmetastatic cause [60–62]. This indication is important, because up to 10% of patients who have NSCLC have an adrenal mass at the time of staging, and about one half to two thirds of these lesions are benign [63,64]. Caution is required in lesions smaller than 1 cm. Specificity of PET for adrenal metastases is high (between 80% and 100%), but some false-positive lesions have been described.

The evaluation of bone metastases in NSCLC by PET has a sensitivity at least equal to that of Technetium-99m bone scan (about 90%) but has a better specificity [65–69], 98% versus 61% in one study [65]. Caution, however, is required with distal

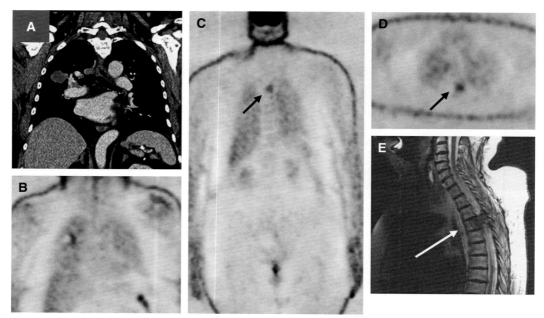

Fig. 5. (*A, B*) The patient has large cell lung cancer in the right upper lobe. (*C, D*) There is a suspected bone lesion in the thoracic spine (*arrow*). (*E*) Bone CT was equivocal, but MR imaging of the spine confirmed bone and soft tissue metastasis (*arrow*).

lesions (eg, below the knee) that fall outside the field of view of a standard "whole-body" PET acquisition and with osteoblastic lesions, which are more readily seen on Technetium-99m bone scan, as demonstrated in a study of patients who had breast cancer [70]. Because most bone lesions in NSCLC are in the central skeleton, and nearly all are osteolytic, PET scan usually replaces bone scan, except in specific clinical indications.

The standard method for the detection of liver metastases is ultrasonography or CT. There are no specific series on the use of PET in patients who have liver metastases from NSCLC. Some general series on staging NSCLC suggest that PET is more accurate than CT [47,50]. Other series on different types of tumors have reported a nonsignificant difference in sensitivity (93% versus 97%), specificity (75% versus 88%), and accuracy (85% versus 92%) for CT and PET, respectively, in the detection of liver involvement [71,72]. Thus, ultrasonography and CT remain the standard imaging techniques for the liver. Additional diagnostic information is provided by PET combined with CT, namely in the differentiation of hepatic lesions that are indeterminate on conventional imaging [71].

FDG-PET is not sensitive enough to exclude brain metastases, because of the high glucose uptake of normal surrounding brain tissue. MR imaging (or CT) remains the method of choice to stage the brain.

Although some PET images can be considered definite proof of multifocal metastatic disease (Fig. 7), caution always is indicated in solitary extrathoracic PET findings that determine the chances for radical therapy (Fig. 8). In these patients, a confirmatory test, such as needle aspiration cytology of an adrenal gland abnormality or demonstration of osteolysis on bone imaging, is indicated.

Baseline staging: consequences of PET in the work-up of non–small cell lung cancer

Guidance of invasive procedures

In addition to CT, PET is of help in directing tissue-sampling techniques in the staging of lung cancer. This is the case for mediastinoscopy as well as for the more recent ultrasound-guided endoscopic techniques such as esophageal ultrasonography (EUS) or endobronchial ultrasonography (EBUS) with a curved linear array ultrasound transducer (Fig. 9). The advent of endoscopic ultrasonography has allowed imaging beyond the mucosa into the mediastinum.

EUS is performed with an esophageal endoscope that guides the ultrasound image through the esophageal wall toward the mediastinal LN of interest, allowing a controlled fine-needle aspiration (FNA) through the working channel of the endoscope. This technique is particularly interesting for

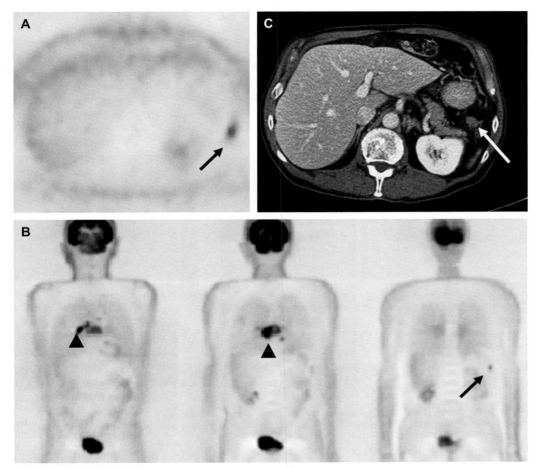

Fig. 6. (*A, B*) The patient had stage IIIB NSCLC (central tumor and contralateral lymph node spread) (*arrowheads*) and an FDG-avid lesion in the left upper abdomen (*arrow*). (*C*) Abdominal CT suggested a colon lesion (*arrow*) that was confirmed to be early colorectal cancer at colonoscopy.

the posterior and inferior mediastinal LNs, which fall outside the reach of mediastinoscopy. A recent review compared CT, PET, and EUS-FNA [30]. The review reported a sensitivity of 57% and a specificity of 82% for CT, of 84% and 89%, respectively, for PET, and of 78% and 71%, respectively, for EUS-FNA. Another series of consecutive patients who had suspected lung cancer on chest radiograph

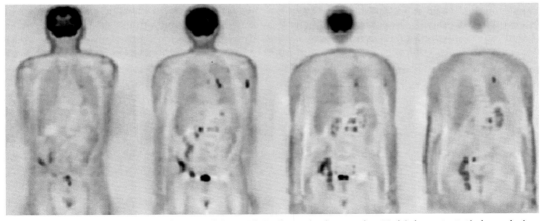

Fig. 7. Adenocarcinoma in the left upper lobe with ipsilateral adenopathy. Multiple metastatic bone lesions.

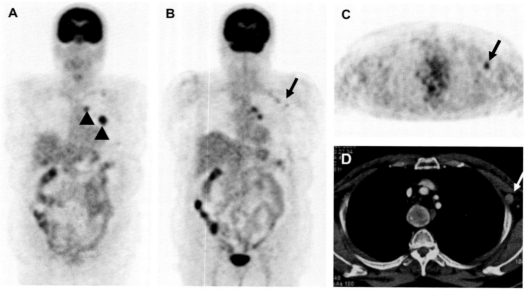

Fig. 8. (*A*) A 71-year-old woman who has left lung tumor with accompanying left para-aortic lymph nodes (*arrowheads*). (*B, C*) FDG-PET also suggested left axillary lymph node metastases (*arrow*). (*D*) CT showed a similar picture. Biopsy revealed inflammatory hydradenitis. With final-stage cT2N2 disease, the patient was a candidate for radical multimodality treatment.

compared CT, PET, and EUS-FNA [73]. PET and EUS-FNA had similar sensitivities (63% versus 68%, respectively) and similar negative predictive values (64% versus 68%, respectively), but EUS-FNA had superior specificity (100%, versus 72% for PET; *P* = .004). Another series compared the accuracy of EUS-FNA of the posterior/inferior mediastinal LN stations in patients who had had a positive PET or CT scan. The accuracy of EUS-FNA was 97%, whereas the accuracy of PET was only 50% [74]. A smaller series concentrated on EUS-FNA in patients who had positive mediastinal LNs on PET. The sensitivity, specificity, negative predictive value, positive predictive value, and accuracy of EUS-FNA in analyzing PET-positive nodes were 93%, 100%, 80%, 100%, and 94%, respectively [75].

EBUS can be performed with a bronchoscope, allowing needle aspiration of superior mediastinal, subcarinal, and hilar LNs under direct ultrasound vision (EBUS-controlled transbronchial needle aspiration [TBNA]). Only one series is available so far comparing EBUS-controlled TBNA, PET only, and thoracic CT in the detection of mediastinal and hilar LN metastasis in patients who have lung cancer considered for surgical resection. The series reported a sensitivity of 92.3%, a specificity of 100%, and diagnostic accuracy of 98% for EBUS-TBNA; of 80%, of 70.1%, and 72.5%, respectively, for PET; and of 76.9%, 55.3%, and 60.8%, respectively, for CT [76].

Impact on overall stage and management

Noninvasive lung cancer staging was improved substantially by the use of PET. The most exciting feature of PET is that it gives a reasonably cancer-specific imaging of the entire patient in one single, noninvasive test. Apart from the information on the probability of malignancy in the primary lesion, the technique is can stage both intra- and extra-thoracic sites in one examination, with a better accuracy than conventional imaging and thus with a potential impact on stage designation and therapeutic decision.

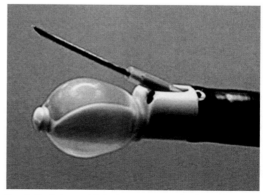

Fig. 9. Endobronchial ultrasonography bronchoscope with a curved linear array ultrasound transducer allowing real-time fine-needle aspiration.

For preoperative mediastinal LN staging, PET has become the most accurate noninvasive diagnostic test. The additional use of PET in preoperative or preradiation therapy staging led to a stage shift in about half (range, 19%–62%) of patients staged with conventional CT. The changes mostly involved upstaging (range, 12%–56%), less frequently involved downstaging, and were related mainly to the detection of unexpected distant lesions by PET (range, 10%–36%) [48,51–54,58,77–80]. In 19% to 46% of cases, the addition of PET imaging also resulted in a change of treatment plan, that is, a change in treatment intent (curative versus palliative), in treatment modality (surgery versus radiotherapy), or in treatment planning (eg, field of radiotherapy) [42,46,48,51,53,54,58,77–80].

A randomized trial addressed whether PET can reduce the number of futile thoracotomies. In the Pet in Lung cancer Staging (PLUS) trial, PET added to conventional imaging strikingly reduced the number of futile thoracotomies in patients who had potentially resectable NSCLC [59]. There was a significant reduction of futile thoracotomies, from 41% in the group assessed with conventional imaging alone to 21% in the group assessed with conventional imaging plus PET, irrespective of clinical stage. Furthermore, PET did not decrease nonfutile thoracotomies (44% versus 41%), because PET improved identification of patients who would benefit from thoracotomy. On the other hand, the recent prospective POORT study illustrated that the use of PET immediately after first presentation did not reduce the overall number of diagnostic tests in comparison with traditional work-up [81]. This study had an inherent limitation in the protocol design: PET scans were not read in conjunction with CT, an approach that is known to improve the accuracy of both tests.

Small cell lung cancer

In contrast to the multitude of data on PET in NSCLC, there are far fewer studies of its accuracy in small cell lung cancer (SCLC) [82–87]. There are several possible reasons. First, SCLC now represents only 15% to 20% of all lung cancers. Second, it is a tumor with early spread into distant sites, thereby obviating the need for PET in many patients. For that reason, patients who have SCLC often are categorized as having limited disease (LD) or extensive disease (ED). According to the consensus definition of the International Association for the Study of Lung Cancer (IASLC), patients who have a tumor confined to one hemithorax including contralateral hilar and supraclavicular nodes have LD [88] These patients are candidates for radical concurrent chemoradiotherapy [89].

Patients who have ED have palliative chemotherapy only.

Regarding the main goal of baseline SCLC staging—the distinction between LD and ED—one prospective study examined how often PET detected ED SCLC in patients considered to have LD based on conventional staging [90]. PET correctly upstaged 2 of 24 patients to ED. PET also correctly depicted all tumor sites in the primary mass and nodal stations. PET impacted the radiotherapy planning by detecting unsuspected locoregional LN metastasis in 6 of 24 patients.

In the largest study to date, 91 patients who had SCLC underwent conventional staging including cranial MR imaging or CT and FDG-PET [91]. In 14 patients, PET caused a stage migration, correctly upstaging 10 patients to ED and downstaging 3 patients to LD. PET was significantly superior to CT in detecting extrathoracic metastases except for the brain.

Restaging after induction therapy

One of the greatest challenges in noninvasive staging is the optimal reassessment of tumor response after induction therapy, including the pathologic response in the primary tumor as well as the downstaging of mediastinal LNs.

The assessment of the tumor response to induction treatment usually is performed on CT imaging. A reduction in tumor volume after induction therapy is considered a predictor of pathologic tumor response. Definitive pathologic assessment of the primary tumor or mediastinal LNs, however, sometimes shows pathologic complete response or mediastinal downstaging, despite the absence of radiologic changes in the tumor volume after induction therapy. Because FDG preferentially accumulates in viable tumor cells and not in fibrotic or necrotic tissue, a change in FDG uptake on PET after induction therapy is considered a better parameter for response evaluation and restaging after induction chemotherapy.

The clinical experience with PET for the detection of residual primary tumor or mediastinal LN involvement after induction therapy for operable NSCLC is rapidly increasing. Eleven studies, most with a small number of patients, are available [92–102].

Some of these studies demonstrated that a repeat PET after induction therapy accurately detects viable tissue in the primary tumor with a sensitivity ranging from 67% to 97% [92,93,97,98]. The presence of false-positive findings in the primary tumor, especially after chemoradiotherapy, hampers the usefulness of PET scan for response evaluation after induction therapy, however.

PET is less sensitive in staging LNs after induction treatment than in the untreated patient. Six mediastinal restaging studies yield a lower sensitivity of PET, ranging from 20% to 71% [92–94,96,97]. Three prospective studies have been performed on a homogeneous group of patients who had pathology-confirmed baseline stage III NSCLC [95–97]. PET after induction chemotherapy for stage IIIA-N2 NSCLC had a sensitivity of 71% in the detection of persistent mediastinal LN disease in one group [96]; a sensitivity of 58% was reported in a study with chemoradiotherapy induction [97]. In the three other studies [92–94], only a minority of the patients had baseline pathology-proven mediastinal LN involvement. One study is difficult to interpret, because only a minority of patients underwent a baseline PET [92]. A second small, prospective study with 34 patients receiving induction chemotherapy for stage IB-IIIA NSCLC reported a disappointing sensitivity of only 50% for detection of malignant LN involvement in general but a surprisingly accurate prediction of the paratracheal N2 LN status with a sensitivity of 100% [93]. In the third small, prospective study with 25 patients, PET after induction chemotherapy for stage IB-IIIA NSCLC had a sensitivity of only 20% for pathologic mediastinal involvement [94]. Although metabolic imaging has the potential of improving the restaging of the primary tumor and mediastinum after induction therapy, its clinical role has not been well defined by the currently available data. More and larger prospective data are needed.

Very recently, two prospective trials studied the role of fusion PET-CT in stage IIIA-N2 NSCLC. A LLCG study compared the role of integrated PET-CT and re-mediastinoscopy to assess pathologic staging after induction chemotherapy. The results of re-mediastinoscopy were disappointing, but the sensitivity and specificity of integrated PET-CT were better than that of visually compared PET and CT images (77% and 92%, respectively) (Fig. 10) [96,99]. Similar results were found by Cerfolio and colleagues [100], although the nature of the study was different. Fusion PET-CT and repeated CT were compared with definitive pathologic staging after induction chemoradiotherapy. A statistical significance in direct comparison was achieved in favor of integrated PET-CT.

Pitfalls in staging lung cancer with PET

False-negative findings

A critical mass of metabolically active malignant cells is required for PET detection of a neoplastic site. LN and distant staging results with PET should be interpreted with caution in tumors with decreased FDG uptake, such as very well-differentiated adenocarcinoma, bronchoalveolar carcinoma, or carcinoid tumors. Furthermore, factors inherent to the technique, such as perivenous FDG injection, or high baseline glucose serum levels should be taken into account.

False-positive findings

FDG uptake is not specific for malignancy, and false-positive findings can occur in any part of the body that has increased glucose metabolic activity (Box 1). Infections and inflammatory conditions, such as bacterial pneumonia [103] or pyogenic

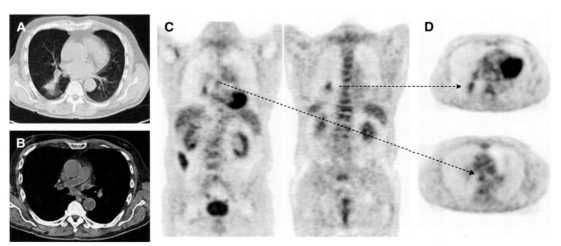

Fig. 10. A patient who has stage IIIA-N2 disease. After induction chemotherapy, (A) the primary tumor in the right lung and (B) the subcarinal adenopathy have decreased in size. On (C) coronal and (D) transaxial PET images, moderate FDG uptake is still present in the primary and in the subcarinal space. Endoscopic needle aspiration confirmed persistent N2 disease.

Box 1: Possible false-positive findings on PET for lung cancer

Infections
(Postobstructive) pneumonia
Mycobacterial or fungal infection

Inflammatory conditions
Granulomatous disorders (eg, sarcoidosis, Wegener disease)
Chronic nonspecific lymphadenitis
(Rheumatoid) arthritis
Occupational (anthracosilicosis)
Reflux esophagitis
Nonspecific (bronchiectasis, organizing pneumonia)

Iatrogenic causes
Radiation esophagitis
Radiation pneumonitis
Bone marrow hyperplasia after chemotherapy
Colony-stimulating factors
Invasive procedures (lymph node or lung biopsy; thoracocentesis; chest tube)

Physiologic causes
Muscle activity
Unilateral vocal cord activity (paralysis other side)
Aortic wall (atherosclerotic plaque)
Brown fat

Benign mass lesions
Salivary gland adenoma–Whartin tumor
Thyroid adenoma
Adrenal adenoma
Colorectal dysplastic polyp

abscess, or aspergillosis and granulomatous diseases, such as active sarcoidosis [104], tuberculosis, histoplasmosis, coccidiomycosis, Wegener's disease, and coal miner's lung, are the most common conditions. In these lesions, the FDG uptake has been attributed to an increase in granulocyte or macrophage activity [105]. Recently, brown fat gained attention as a possible cause of benign FDG uptake. Brown fat usually has a bilateral and symmetric distribution but may be asymmetric and focal. Because this uptake may occur in regions of potential malignant LN spread (cervical, supraclavicular, axillary, mediastinal, and abdominal regions), the differential diagnosis may be difficult when PET images are interpreted without the aid of CT images. In most instances, correlation with CT images, preferably by PET-CT fusion images, can resolve the problem [106].

References

[1] Schrevens L, Lorent N, Dooms C, et al. The role of PET-scan in diagnosis, staging and management of non-small cell lung cancer. Oncologist 2004;9:633–43.

[2] Vansteenkiste J, Fischer BM, Dooms C, et al. Positron-emission tomography in prognostic and therapeutic assessment of lung cancer: systematic review. Lancet Oncol 2004;5:531–40.

[3] Mountain CF. Revisions in the international system for staging lung cancer. Chest 1997;111(6): 1710–7.

[4] Naruke T, Suemasu K, Ishikawa S. Lymph node mapping and curability at various levels of metastasis in resected lung cancer. J Thorac Cardiovasc Surg 1978;76:832–7.

[5] American Thoracic Society (ATS). Clinical staging of primary lung cancer. Am Rev Respir Dis 1983;127:1–11.

[6] Mountain CF, Dresler CM. Regional lymph node classification for lung cancer staging. Chest 1997;111(6):1718–23.

[7] Vansteenkiste J, Dooms C, Becker H, et al. Multimodality treatment of stage III non-small cell lung cancer: staging procedures. Eur J Cancer 2005;3(Suppl 3):7–19.

[8] Arriagada R, Bergman B, Dunant A, et al. for the International Adjuvant Lung Cancer Trial Collaborative Group. Cisplatin-based adjuvant chemotherapy in patients with completely resected non-small cell lung cancer. N Engl J Med 2004;350:351–60.

[9] Jett JR, Scott WJ, Rivera MP, et al. Guidelines on treatment of stage IIIB non-small cell lung cancer. Chest 2003;123(Suppl 1):221S–5S.

[10] Vansteenkiste J, De Leyn P, Deneffe G, et al. Present status of induction treatment for N2 non-small cell lung cancer: a review. Eur J Cardiothorac Surg 1998;13:1–12.

[11] Rosell R, Gomez Codina J, Camps C, et al. A randomized trial comparing preoperative chemotherapy plus surgery with surgery alone in patients with non-small-cell lung cancer. N Engl J Med 1994;330:153–8.

[12] Betticher DC, Hsu Schmitz SF, Totsch M, et al. Mediastinal lymph node clearance after docetaxel-cisplatin neoadjuvant chemotherapy is prognostic of survival in patients with stage IIIA pN2 non-small cell lung cancer: a multicenter phase II trial. J Clin Oncol 2003;21:1752–9.

[13] Lorent N, De Leyn P, Lievens Y, et al. Long-term survival of surgically staged IIIA-N2 non-small cell lung cancer treated with surgical combined modality approach: analysis of a 7-year experience. Ann Oncol 2004;15:1645–53.

[14] Vansteenkiste JF, Vandebroek JE, Nackaerts KL, et al. Clinical benefit response in advanced non-small cell lung cancer. A multicenter prospective randomized phase III study of single agent gemcitabine versus cisplatin-vindesine. Ann Oncol 2001;12:1221–30.

[15] Numico G, Russi E, Merlano M. Best supportive care in non-small cell lung cancer: is there a role for radiotherapy and chemotherapy? Lung Cancer 2001;32:213–26.

[16] Bittner RC, Felix R. Magnetic resonance (MR) imaging of the chest: state-of-the-art. Eur Respir J 1998;11:1392–404.

[17] Glazer HS, Kaiser LR, Anderson DJ, et al. Indeterminate mediastinal invasion in bronchogenic carcinoma: CT evaluation. Radiology 1989;173(1):37–42.

[18] Kameda K, Adachi S, Kono M. Detection of T-factor in lung cancer using magnetic resonance imaging and computed tomography. J Thorac Imaging 1988;3(2):73–80.

[19] Izbicki JR, Thetter O, Karg O, et al. Accuracy of computed tomographic scan and surgical assessment for staging of bronchial carcinoma. A prospective study. J Thorac Cardiovasc Surg 1992;104(2):413–20.

[20] Hierholzer J, Luo L, Bittner RC, et al. MRI and CT in the differential diagnosis of pleural disease. Chest 2000;118(3):604–9.

[21] Pearlberg JL, Sandler MA, Beute GH, et al. Limitations of CT in evaluation of neoplasms involving chest wall. J Comput Assist Tomogr 1987;11(2):290–3.

[22] Lardinois D, Weder W, Hany TF, et al. Staging of non-small cell lung cancer with integrated positron-emission tomography and computed tomography. N Engl J Med 2003;348:2500–7.

[23] De Wever W, Ceyssens S, Mortelmans L, et al. Additional value of PET-CT in the staging of lung cancer: comparison with CT alone, PET alone and visual correlation of PET and CT. Eur Radiol 2006.

[24] Erasmus JJ, McAdams HP, Rossi SE, et al. FDG PET of pleural effusions in patients with non-small cell lung cancer. AJR Am J Roentgenol 2000;175:245–9.

[25] Gupta NC, Rogers JS, Graeber GM, et al. Clinical role of F-18 fluorodeoxyglucose positron emission tomography imaging in patients with lung cancer and suspected malignant pleural effusion. Chest 2002;122:1918–24.

[26] Schaffler GJ, Wolf G, Schoellnast H, et al. Non-small cell lung cancer: evaluation of pleural abnormalities on CT scans with 18F FDG PET. Radiology 2004;231:858–65.

[27] Shim SS, Lee KS, Kim BT, et al. Integrated PET/CT and the dry pleural dissemination of peripheral adenocarcinoma of the lung: diagnostic implications. J Comput Assist Tomogr 2006;30:70–6.

[28] Martini N, Kris MG, Ginsberg RJ. The role of multimodality therapy in locoregional non-small cell lung cancer. Surg Oncol Clin N Am 1997;6:769–91.

[29] Dillemans B, Deneffe G, Verschakelen J, et al. Value of computed tomography and mediastinoscopy in preoperative evaluation of mediastinal nodes in non-small cell lung cancer. Eur J Cardiothorac Surg 1994;8:37–42.

[30] Toloza EM, Harpole L, McCrory DC. Noninvasive staging of non-small cell lung cancer: a review of the current evidence. Chest 2003;123 (Suppl 1):137S–46S.

[31] Vansteenkiste JF, Stroobants SG, De Leyn PR, et al. Lymph node staging in non-small cell lung cancer with FDG-PET scan: a prospective study on 690 lymph node stations from 68 patients. J Clin Oncol 1998;16:2142–9.

[32] Dwamena BA, Sonnad SS, Angobaldo JO, et al. Metastases from non-small cell lung cancer: mediastinal staging in the 1990s. Meta-analytic comparison of PET and CT. Radiology 1999; 213:530–6.

[33] Fischer BM, Mortensen J, Hojgaard L. Positron emission tomography in the diagnosis and staging of lung cancer: a systematic, quantitative review. Lancet Oncol 2001;2:659–66.

[34] Hellwig D, Ukena D, Paulsen F, et al. Meta-analysis of the efficacy of positron emission tomography with F-18-fluorodeoxyglucose in lung tumors. Basis for discussion of the German Consensus Conference on PET in Oncology 2000 (in German). Pneumologie 2001;55: 367–77.

[35] Gould MK, Kuschner WG, Rydzak CE, et al. Test performance of positron emission tomography and computed tomography for mediastinal staging in patients with non-small cell lung cancer: a meta-analysis. Ann Intern Med 2003; 139:879–92.

[36] Gupta NC, Graeber GM, Bishop HA. Comparative efficacy of positron emission tomography with fluorodeoxyglucose in evaluation of small (3 cm) lymph node lesions. Chest 2000;117(3): 773–8.

[37] Vansteenkiste JF. FDG-PET for lymph node staging in NSCLC: a major step forward, but beware of the pitfalls. [editorial]. Lung Cancer 2005;47: 151–3.

[38] Takamochi K, Yoshida J, Murakami K, et al. Pitfalls in lymph node staging with positron emission tomography in non-small cell lung cancer patients. Lung Cancer 2005;47:235–42.

[39] Vansteenkiste JF, De Leyn PR, Deneffe GJ, et al. Survival and prognostic factors in resected N2 non-small cell lung cancer: a study of 140 cases. The Leuven Lung Cancer Group. Ann Thorac Surg 1997;63:1441–50.

[40] Bollen EC, Theunissen PH, Van Duin CJ, et al. Clinical significance of intranodal and extranodal growth in lymph node metastases of non-small cell lung cancer. Scand J Thorac Cardiovasc Surg 1994;28:97–102.

[41] Vansteenkiste JF, Stroobants SG, De Leyn PR, et al. Mediastinal lymph node staging with FDG-PET scan in patients with potentially operable non-small cell lung cancer: a prospective analysis of 50 cases. Chest 1997;112:1480–6.

[42] Weng E, Tran L, Rege S, et al. Accuracy and clinical impact of mediastinal lymph node staging with FDG-PET imaging in potentially resectable lung cancer. Am J Clin Oncol 2000;23(1): 47–52.

[43] Fritscher-Ravens A, Bohuslavizki KH, Brandt L, et al. Mediastinal lymph node involvement in

potentially resectable lung cancer: comparison of CT, positron emission tomography, and endoscopic ultrasonography with and without fine-needle aspiration. Chest 2003;123: 442–51.

[44] Quint LE, Tummala S, Brisson LJ, et al. Distribution of distant metastases from newly diagnosed non- small cell lung cancer. Ann Thorac Surg 1996;62(1):246–50.

[45] Pantel K, Izbicki J, Passlick B, et al. Frequency and prognostic significance of isolated tumour cells in bone marrow of patients with non-small cell lung cancer without overt metastases. Lancet 1996;347(9002):649–53.

[46] Lewis P, Griffin S, Marsden P, et al. Whole-body 18F-fluorodeoxyglucose positron emission tomography in preoperative evaluation of lung cancer. Lancet 1994;344:1265–6.

[47] Valk PE, Pounds TR, Hopkins DM, et al. Staging non-small cell lung cancer by whole-body positron emission tomographic imaging. Ann Thorac Surg 1995;60(6):1573–81.

[48] Bury T, Dowlati A, Paulus P, et al. Whole-body 18FDG positron emission tomography in the staging of non-small cell lung cancer. Eur Respir J 1997;10:2529–34.

[49] Weder W, Schmid RA, Bruchhaus H, et al. Detection of extrathoracic metastases by positron emission tomography in lung cancer. Ann Thorac Surg 1998;66(3):886–92.

[50] Marom EM, McAdams HP, Erasmus JJ, et al. Staging non-small cell lung cancer with whole-body PET. Radiology 1999;212(3): 803–9.

[51] Saunders CA, Dussek JE, O'Doherty MJ, et al. Evaluation of fluorine-18-fluorodeoxyglucose whole body positron emission tomography imaging in the staging of lung cancer. Ann Thorac Surg 1999;67(3):790–7.

[52] Pieterman RM, Van Putten JW, Meuzelaar JJ, et al. Preoperative staging of non-small cell lung cancer with positron emission tomography. N Engl J Med 2000;343:254–61.

[53] Mac Manus MP, Hicks RJ, Matthews JP, et al. High rate of detection of unsuspected distant metastases by PET in apparent stage III non-small cell lung cancer: implications for radical radiation therapy. Int J Radiat Oncol Biol Phys 2001;50:287–93.

[54] Hicks RJ, Kalff V, Mac Manus MP, et al. 18F-FDG PET provides high-impact and powerful prognostic stratification in staging newly diagnosed non-small cell lung cancer. J Nucl Med 2001;42:1596–604.

[55] Eschmann SM, Friedel G, Paulsen F, et al. FDG PET for staging of advanced non-small cell lung cancer prior to neoadjuvant radio-chemotherapy. Eur J Nucl Med Mol Imaging 2002;29: 804–8.

[56] Vesselle H, Pugsley JM, Vallieres E, et al. The impact of fluorodeoxyglucose F18 positron emission tomography on the surgical staging of non-small cell lung cancer. J Thorac Cardiovasc Surg 2002;124:511–9.

[57] Stroobants S, Dhoore I, Dooms C, et al. Additional value of whole-body fluorodeoxyglucose positron emission tomography in the detection of distant metastases of non-small cell lung cancer. Clin Lung Cancer 2003;4:242–7.

[58] Hoekstra CJ, Stroobants SG, Hoekstra OS, et al. The value of [18F]fluoro-2-deoxy-D-glucose positron emission tomography in the selection of patients with stage IIIA-N2 non-small cell lung cancer for combined modality treatment. Lung Cancer 2003;39:151–7.

[59] Van Tinteren H, Hoekstra OS, Smit EF, et al. Effectiveness of positron emission tomography in the preoperative assessment of patients with suspected non-small cell lung cancer: the PLUS multicentre randomised trial. Lancet 2002;359:1388–93.

[60] Erasmus JJ, Patz EF, McAdams HP, et al. Evaluation of adrenal masses in patients with bronchogenic carcinoma using 18F-fluorodeoxyglucose positron emission tomography. AJR Am J Roentgenol 1997;168(5):1357–60.

[61] Boland GW, Goldberg MA, Lee MJ, et al. Indeterminate adrenal mass in patients with cancer: evaluation at PET with 2-[F-18]-fluoro-2-deoxy-D-glucose. Radiology 1995;194(1):131–4.

[62] Yun M, Kim W, Alnafisi N, et al. 18F-FDG PET in characterizing adrenal lesions detected on CT or MRI. J Nucl Med 2001;42:1795–7.

[63] Oliver TW, Bernardino ME, Miller JI, et al. Isolated adrenal masses in non-small cell bronchogenic carcinoma. Radiology 1984;153(1):217–8.

[64] Ettinghausen SE, Burt ME. Prospective evaluation of unilateral adrenal masses in patients with operable non-small cell lung cancer. J Clin Oncol 1991;9(8):1462–6.

[65] Bury T, Barreto A, Daenen F, et al. Fluorine-18 deoxyglucose positron emission tomography for the detection of bone metastases in patients with non-small cell lung cancer. Eur J Nucl Med 1998;25(9):1244–7.

[66] Hsia TC, Shen YY, Yen RF, et al. Comparing whole body 18F-2-deoxyglucose positron emission tomography and technetium-99m methylene diophosphate bone scan to detect bone metastases in patients with non-small cell lung cancer. Neoplasma 2002;49:267–71.

[67] Gayed I, Vu T, Johnson M, et al. Comparison of bone and 2-deoxy-2-[18F]fluoro-D-glucose positron emission tomography in the evaluation of bony metastases in lung cancer. Mol Imaging Biol 2003;5:26–31.

[68] Cheran SK, Herndon JE, Patz EF. Comparison of whole-body FDG-PET to bone scan for detection of bone metastases in patients with a new diagnosis of lung cancer. Lung Cancer 2004;44:317–25.

[69] Kao CH, Hsieh JF, Tsai SC, et al. Comparison and discrepancy of 18F-2-deoxyglucose positron emission tomography and Tc-99m MDP

bone scan to detect bone metastases. Anticancer Res 2000;20(3B):2189–92.

[70] Cook GJ, Houston S, Rubens R, et al. Detection of bone metastases in breast cancer by 18FDG PET: differing metabolic activity in osteoblastic and osteolytic lesions. J Clin Oncol 1998; 16(10):3375–9.

[71] Hustinx R, Paulus P, Jacquet N, et al. Clinical evaluation of whole-body 18F-fluorodeoxyglucose positron emission tomography in the detection of liver metastases. Ann Oncol 1998; 9(4):397–401.

[72] Delbeke D, Martin WH, Sandler MP, et al. Evaluation of benign vs malignant hepatic lesions with positron emission tomography. Arch Surg 1998;133(5):510–5.

[73] Fritscher-Ravens A, Davidson BL, Hauber HP, et al. Endoscopic ultrasound, positron emission tomography, and computerized tomography for lung cancer. Am J Respir Crit Care Med 2003;168:1293–7.

[74] Eloubeidi MA, Cerfolio RJ, Chen VK, et al. Endoscopic ultrasound-guided fine needle aspiration of mediastinal lymph node in patients with suspected lung cancer after positron emission tomography and computed tomography scans. Ann Thorac Surg 2005;79:263–8.

[75] Annema JT, Hoekstra OS, Smit EF, et al. Towards a minimally invasive staging strategy in NSCLC: analysis of PET positive mediastinal lesions by EUS-FNA. Lung Cancer 2004;44: 53–60.

[76] Yasufuku K, Nakajima T, Motoori K, et al. Comparison of endobronchial ultrasound, positron emission tomography, and CT for lymph node staging of lung cancer. Chest 2006;130(3): 710–8.

[77] Vanuytsel LJ, Vansteenkiste JF, Stroobants SG, et al. The impact of (18)F-fluoro-2-deoxy-D-glucose positron emission tomography (FDG-PET) lymph node staging on the radiation treatment volumes in patients with non-small cell lung cancer. Radiother Oncol 2000;55:317–24.

[78] Kalff V, Hicks RJ, Mac Manus M, et al. Clinical impact of (18)F-fluorodeoxyglucose positron emission tomography in patients with non-small cell lung cancer: A prospective study. J Clin Oncol 2001;19:111–8.

[79] Changlai SP, Tsai SC, Chou MC, et al. Whole body 18F–2-deoxyglucose positron emission tomography to restage non-small cell lung cancer. Oncol Rep 2001;8:337–9.

[80] Dizendorf EV, Baumert BG, Von Schulthess GK, et al. Impact of whole-body 18F-FDG PET on staging and managing patients for radiation therapy. J Nucl Med 2003;44:24–9.

[81] Herder GJ, Kramer H, Hoekstra OS, et al. Traditional versus up-front [18F] fluorodeoxyglucose positron emission tomography staging of non-small cell lung cancer: a Dutch cooperative randomized study. J Clin Oncol 2006;24(12): 1800–6.

[82] Schumacher T, Brink I, Mix M, et al. FDG-PET imaging for the staging and follow-up of small cell lung cancer. Eur J Nucl Med 2001;28: 483–8.

[83] Chin R, McCain TW, Miller AA, et al. Whole body FDG-PET for the evaluation and staging of small cell lung cancer: a preliminary study. Lung Cancer 2002;37:1–6.

[84] Shen YY, Shiau YC, Wang JJ, et al. Whole-body 18F-2-deoxyglucose positron emission tomography in primary staging small cell lung cancer. Anticancer Res 2002;22:1257–64.

[85] Zhao DS, Valdivia AY, Li Y, et al. 18F-fluorodeoxyglucose positron emission tomography in small cell lung cancer. Semin Nucl Med 2002;32:272–5.

[86] Kamel EM, Zwahlen D, Wyss MT, et al. Whole-body 18F-FDG PET improves the management of patients with small cell lung cancer. J Nucl Med 2003;44:1911–7.

[87] Blum R, Mac Manus MP, Rischin D, et al. Impact of positron emission tomography on the management of patients with small cell lung cancer: preliminary experience. Am J Clin Oncol 2004;27:164–71.

[88] Micke P, Faldum A, Metz T, et al. Staging small cell lung cancer: Veterans Administration Lung Study Group versus International Association for the Study of Lung Cancer—what limits limited disease? Lung Cancer 2002;37:271–6.

[89] De Ruysscher D, Vansteenkiste J. Chest radiotherapy in limited stage small cell lung cancer: facts, questions, prospects. Radiother Oncol 2000;55:1–9.

[90] Bradley JD, Dehdashti F, Mintun MA, et al. Positron emission tomography in limited-stage small cell lung cancer: a prospective study. J Clin Oncol 2004;22:3248–54.

[91] Brink I, Schumacher T, Mix M, et al. Impact of 18F-FDG-PET on the primary staging of small cell lung cancer. Eur J Nucl Med Mol Imaging 2005;31:1614–20.

[92] Akhurst T, Downey RJ, Ginsberg MS, et al. An initial experience with FDG-PET in the imaging of residual disease after induction therapy for lung cancer. Ann Thorac Surg 2002;73:259–66.

[93] Cerfolio RJ, Ojha B, Mukherjee S, et al. Positron emission tomography scanning with 2-fluoro-2-deoxy-d- glucose as a predictor of response of neoadjuvant treatment for non-small cell carcinoma. J Thorac Cardiovasc Surg 2003; 125:938–44.

[94] Port JL, Kent MS, Korst RJ, et al. Positron emission tomography scanning poorly predicts response to preoperative chemotherapy in non-small cell lung cancer. Ann Thorac Surg 2004; 77:254–9.

[95] Vansteenkiste JF, Stroobants SG, De Leyn PR, et al. Potential use of FDG-PET scan after induction chemotherapy in surgically staged IIIA-N2 non-small cell lung cancer: a prospective pilot study. Ann Oncol 1998;9:1193–8.

[96] Vansteenkiste J, Stroobants S, Hoekstra C, et al. 18fluoro-2-deoxyglucose positron emission tomography (PET) in the assessment of induction chemotherapy (IC) in stage IIIA-N2 NSCLC: a multi-center prospective study. Proc Am Soc Clin Oncol 2001;20:313A.

[97] Ryu JS, Choi NC, Fischman AJ, et al. FDG-PET in staging and restaging non-small cell lung cancer after neoadjuvant chemoradiotherapy: correlation with histopathology. Lung Cancer 2002;35:179–87.

[98] Choi NC, Fischman AJ, Niemierko A, et al. Dose-response relationship between probability of pathologic tumor control and glucose metabolic rate measured with FDG PET after preoperative chemoradiotherapy in locally advanced non-small cell lung cancer. Int J Radiat Oncol Biol Phys 2002;54:1024–35.

[99] De Leyn P, Stroobants S, De Wever W, et al. Prospective comparative study of integrated positron emission tomography-computed tomography compared with remediastinoscopy in the assessment of residual mediastinal lymph node disease after induction chemotherapy for mediastinoscopy proven stage IIIA-N2 non-small cell lung cancer: A Leuven Lung Cancer Group study. J Clin Oncol 2006;24: 3333–9.

[100] Cerfolio RJ, Bryant AS, Ojha B. Restaging patients with N2 (stage IIIa) non-small cell lung cancer after neoadjuvant chemoradiotherapy: a prospective study. J Thorac Cardiovasc Surg 2006;131(6):1229–35.

[101] Hoekstra CJ, Stroobants SG, Smit EF, et al. Prognostic relevance of response evaluation using [18F]-2-fluoro-2-deoxy-D-glucose positron emission tomography in patients with locally advanced non-small cell lung cancer. J Clin Oncol 2005;23:8362–70.

[102] Ohtsuka T, Nomori H, Ebihara A, et al. FDG-PET imaging for lymph node staging and pathologic tumor response after neoadjuvant treatment of non-small cell lung cancer. Ann Thorac Cardiovasc Surg 2006;12(2):89–94.

[103] Kapucu LO, Meltzer CC, Townsend DW, et al. Fluorine-18-fluorodeoxyglucose uptake in pneumonia. J Nucl Med 1998;39(7):1267–9.

[104] Brudin LH, Valind SO, Rhodes CG, et al. Fluorine-18 deoxyglucose uptake in sarcoidosis measured with positron emission tomography. Eur J Nucl Med 1994;21(4):297–305.

[105] Bakheet SM, Saleem M, Powe J, et al. F-18 fluorodeoxyglucose chest uptake in lung inflammation and infection. Clin Nucl Med 2000;25(4): 273–8.

[106] Truong MT, Erasmus JJ, Munden RF, et al. Focal FDG uptake in mediastinal brown fat mimicking malignancy: a potential pitfall resolved on PET/CT. AJR Am J Roentgenol 2004;183: 1127–32.

ELSEVIER
SAUNDERS

RADIOLOGIC
CLINICS
OF NORTH AMERICA

Radiol Clin N Am 45 (2007) 627–638

Impact of PET on Radiation Therapy Planning in Lung Cancer

Michael P. Mac Manus, MD, MRCP, FRCR, FFRRCSI, FRANZCR[a,*],
Rodney J. Hicks, MD, FRACP[b]

Of all the medical disciplines, radiation oncology could well be the clinical specialty most dependent on accurate three-dimensional imaging. Unlike an oncological surgeon who may modify his or her assessment of the extent of disease during an operation, the radiation oncologist is usually reliant on imaging to guide the entire treatment process, albeit supplemented by pathology reports, clinical examination, and other information depending upon the clinical situation. To direct a tumoricidal dose of radiation to a tumor, while sparing normal tissues as much as possible, the precise spatial location of the primary tumor and of tumor-bearing lymph nodes must be appreciated, together with the anatomy of the critical adjacent normal tissues. A perfect radiation therapy (RT) plan would deliver a lethal dose to the tumor and no dose at all to the normal tissues. Such perfection is of course unattainable with the photon beams produced by linear accelerators, although proton beams may provide a closer approximation [1]. Nevertheless, the use of multiple, carefully shaped and modulated photon beams can produce remarkably good results, but only if treatment is directed to precisely the right location in three-dimensional space.

In the last decade or so, rapid improvements in the technology available for RT planning and delivery have occurred and future developments are

This article was previously published in PET Clinics 2006;1:317–28.
[a] Department of Radiation Oncology, Peter MacCallum Cancer Centre, St Andrew's Place, East Melbourne, Vic 3002, Australia
[b] Centre for Molecular Imaging, Peter MacCallum Cancer Centre, 12 Cathedral Place, East Melbourne, Vic 3002, Australia
* Corresponding author.
E-mail address: mmanus@petermac.unimelb.edu.au (M.P. Mac Manus).

doi:10.1016/j.rcl.2007.05.002

likely [2]. Extraordinarily advanced treatment planning systems now allow much more accurate and rapid three-dimensional radiation dose calculations with quantitative volumetric assessment of dose both to tumor and critical normal tissues [3]. This new complexity in dose calculation has been accompanied by an increased ability to accurately deliver ionizing radiation to complex three-dimensional shapes, using linear accelerators with independently controlled multileaf collimators that can dynamically shape the beam of radiation during the course of treatment delivery [4]. New types of highly conformal radiotherapy such as intensity-modulated radiotherapy have become available [5], making it possible to safely escalate the radiation dose without increased toxicity as in prostate cancer [6], or to maintain existing local control rates with reduced toxicity as in head and neck cancer [7], where new parotid-sparing techniques can often avoid permanent xerostomia.

The relationships between increasing radiation dose and tumor control and increasing radiation dose and the probability of a serious complication of treatment are classically described by paired sigmoid curves (**Fig. 1**). The greater the separation between the tumor control and radiation toxicity curves, the more likely the patient is to achieve uncomplicated local "cure" of their tumor. As a result of relative sparing of normal tissues, the newer more highly conformal RT techniques are capable of increasing the "therapeutic ratio." For a given dose of radiation prescribed to control a tumor, the ratio between the probability of tumor control and the probability of a significant complication is increased. Improving the therapeutic ratio is a key goal of research in radiation oncology.

The more highly conformal RT planning methods, with requirements for tight margins around disease sites, depend especially critically on an accurate assessment of the location of tumor sites in relation to the anatomy of normal tissues. The basis for RT planning has long been the CT scan. CT not only provides important three-dimensional anatomic information, but also provides the basis for radiation dosimetry by reconstruction of a three-dimensional electron-density map that is crucial for calculating radiation absorption and scatter. CT will remain the basis for dose calculation in radiation oncology but the information that it can provide about the location of the tumor is often insufficient by itself to accurately guide treatment. To successfully image a neoplastic lesion on CT, there must be sufficient contrast between the lesion and normal tissues. When tumors have similar imaging characteristics to surrounding normal tissues, which is often the case for lesions in the liver or spleen, they may be completely invisible on CT. Consequently, when CT is used to guide curative RT in such cases, geographic miss and ultimate treatment failure may be inevitable. Failure to image the boundary between tumor and atelectatic lung is also a common problem for the radiation oncologist relying on CT for treating lung cancer and may lead to unnecessary irradiation of large volumes of collapsed lung to avoid a geographic miss. Accurate lymph node staging is crucial for treating locoregionally advanced cancers with curative intent [8,9]. CT scanning often performs relatively poorly in this respect too because nodal size is the usual criterion for deciding if tumor is present or absent. Small nodes, negative by CT criteria, often contain tumor and benign reactive

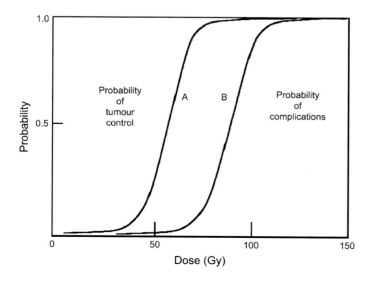

Fig. 1. Typical paired sigmoid dose-response curves for tumor control (*A*) and normal tissue complications (*B*).

lymphadenopathy can commonly give rise to false positives in a variety of cancer sites. A good example of this phenomenon is the notoriously poor sensitivity and specificity reported in numerous clinico-pathological studies of staging the mediastinum in potentially resectable non–small cell lung cancer (NSCLC) [10].

It is fortuitous that, just when dramatic advances in RT technology were being made, a revolution was also occurring in cancer imaging with the advent of clinical PET. Staging with PET, primarily using ^{18}F-fluorodeoxyglucose (FDG) as the tracer, has rapidly acquired a key role in the management of cancers such as NSCLC [11,12], Hodgkin and non-Hodgkin lymphomas [13,14], head and neck cancers, esophageal cancers [15,16], and cervical carcinomas [17,18]. FDG-PET shows great promise in malignant melanoma [19,20], soft tissue sarcoma [21], gastrointestinal cancers [22], and a range of less common neoplasms [23,24]. Other PET tracers have the potential to image lower grade tumors when FDG is less helpful (eg, ^{18}F-labeled fluoroethylcholine in low grade glioma [25]), to identify lesions that are actively proliferating (as with ^{18}F-labeled fluorothymidine [26]), or to identify tumors with radioresistant hypoxic tumors using ^{18}F-labeled misondazole [27].

The new information provided by FDG-PET staging has the potential to immediately improve the results of radical RT by way of better selection of patients. Significantly improved survival has already been demonstrated in patients who have NSCLC selected for radical RT using PET compared with a conventionally staged control group [28], largely because patients who have PET-detected metastases and advanced locoregional disease were denied futile aggressive therapy. Incorporation of PET information into the RT planning process also has the potential to improve targeting of RT by accurately imaging regions of tumor in three dimensions [29]. A revolution in radiotherapy planning is occurring, as ways of incorporating new functional imaging data are continually being sought. In the following sections the role of PET in RT planning will be discussed in more detail.

Importance of imaging in the radiotherapy planning process

The three-dimensional radiotherapy planning process

As discussed above, the primary tool for planning curative RT is cross-sectional imaging with a CT scan. When it has been decided that a patient should receive radical RT, a treatment planning CT scan is performed with the patient in the radiotherapy treatment position with appropriate immobilization devices fitted so that patient positioning

is identical for CT imaging, simulation (if performed separately), and for treatment. CT data are imported into the treatment planning software and areas of tumor are identified and contoured by the radiation oncologist using a pointing device on individual CT slices. This process generates a gross tumor volume (GTV) [30]. Normal tissues are also contoured on individual slices so that volumes of important dose-limiting organs exposed to radiation can be assessed quantitatively.

The volume that actually needs to be treated in radical RT is of course greater than the GTV because additional margins must be applied. These margins allow for a range of factors including microscopic extension of disease beyond the imaged tumor, variability in the accuracy of patient set-up on each day of treatment, and movement of the tumor (eg, with respiration). The margins applied to the GTV are disease and site specific. The volume that the radiation oncologist decides to treat, and that incorporates all of the margins around the GTV, is known as the planning target volume (PTV). The PTV is often an expansion of the GTV, generated automatically by the treatment planning software. An ideal PTV should include all gross and microscopic tumor (or at least microscopic tumor that will not be eliminated by systemic therapy) and be large enough to accommodate movement of the tumor during treatment ("internal target volume" [31]).

The next step in the process is to try to find the optimum arrangement of beams to effectively administer the prescribed radiation dose to the GTV. A variable number of individually shaped and modulated beams is applied from a range of carefully chosen angles. The range of possible solutions to a given planning problem is infinite. An ideal treatment plan would treat all parts of the PTV to the prescribed dose without exposing any healthy normal tissues to radiation. The best available RT treatment plan is one that most closely approximates this ideal and can actually be delivered in a clinical setting. Efforts are made to ensure that the inevitable dose delivered to normal tissues is "dumped" in regions where it will do least harm.

The most important step in the process, and upon which all subsequent steps depend, is the determination of the GTV. If the location of gross tumor in three-dimensional space is not accurately known and a geographic miss occurs, then treatment will be a toxic and futile exercise. Incorporation of PET into the treatment planning process has the potential to make determination of the GTV much more accurate and therefore reduce the risk of futile therapy. It is acknowledged that PET information is far from perfect. Yet for many tumor types, PET provides such a significant increase in accuracy of assessment of tumor extent that failure to use it, if available, would mean denying the patient the best possible treatment plan.

Incorporation of PET information into radiation therapy planning

In the years since the introduction of clinical PET, its importance as a tool for RT planning has become increasingly recognized. Manufacturers have become aware of the need to accommodate the ability to import and display PET information in radiotherapy planning systems. They have produced systems of increasing utility and sophistication, with the most up-to-date systems capable of allowing seamless integration of PET-CT information into the RT contouring workstation. When PET and CT imaging are combined for radiotherapy planning, the aim is to produce a biological target volume [32], incorporating all available structural and functional imaging. For lung cancer and several other malignancies, treatment of the biological target volume represents the best target for high-dose irradiation that we can currently define.

Visual incorporation of PET data into treatment planning

When clinical PET first became available to oncologists, there were no readily available means for incorporating PET information directly into the treatment planning process. Typically, PET and diagnostic CT images were simply displayed side by side on a light box and the radiation oncologist would visually incorporate the PET information when contouring the GTV. For example, if an axillary lymph node was well visualized on the planning CT and was considered uninvolved by size criteria (usually short axis diameter less than 1 cm), it would not normally be contoured as part of the GTV. If the same node, however, was identified as being FDG-avid on a PET scan and was considered to contain tumor, the node would be contoured as part of the GTV despite being negative on size criteria. In our own early prospective lung cancer study, we used this method to incorporate PET into the planning process, without any form of image coregistration. This method works quite well for small anatomically discrete structures that are easily seen on CT, but it is not a good method for helping to delineate the boundaries of larger tumors where the margins are not well imaged on CT, such as the interface between a lung tumor and atelectasis. For that purpose it was necessary to devise some method for displaying PET and CT information simultaneously within the treatment planning software.

Coregistration of separately acquired PET and CT images for treatment planning

To make full use of the three-dimensional imaging information contained in the PET scan, a number of methods were tried at different institutions before manufacturers provided commercial software and hardware solutions to make the process easy. At our own center and at other centers, in-house methods were developed for the purpose of importing PET information into the radiotherapy treatment planning system. We developed a system that used fiducial markers that were applied to the patient at separate CT and PET image acquisitions [33]. For both scans, patients were positioned identically by radiation therapists using lasers installed in both the CT and PET suites. Phantom studies showed that the method was highly reproducible and could be used in clinical practice. Digital imaging and communications in medicine PET information was imported into the radiotherapy planning system (Cadplan, Varian Medical Systems Inc., Palo Alto, California) and displayed side by side with the corresponding CT image, using software developed at our own institution. This proved highly successful in practice but, with the installation of our first combined PET/CT scanner, it has since been entirely superseded.

PET/CT for treatment planning

The optimum dataset for radiotherapy planning is provided by a modern combined PET/CT scanner. PET and CT images are acquired on the same gantry, without the need for repositioning the patient. This represents a major advance on older methods. PET/CT is not available at all centers and many radiation oncologists must rely on CT and PET images obtained at separate acquisitions as described above. Modern treatment planning systems such as Focalease (Computerized Medical Systems Inc., St. Louis, Missouri) and Pinnacle (Philips Medical Systems, Eindhoven, The Netherlands) allow seamless transfer of PET/CT data into the contouring workspace and provide a wide range of options for display of fused PET and CT images. Fig. 2 shows a PET/CT scanner (Discovery LS; GE Medical Systems, Milwaukee, WI) in use at our institution, illustrating the flat couch top and laser system essential for accurate patient positioning for radiotherapy planning. Fig. 3 shows a typical screenshot of a patient who has lung cancer undergoing radiotherapy planning, using Focalsim (Computerized Medical Systems Inc.).

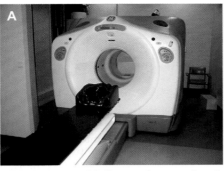
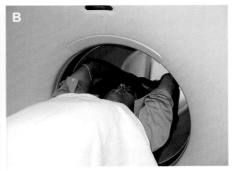

Fig. 2. (*A*) PET/CT scanner with flat couch top and patient-positioning device for lung cancer. (*B*) Positioning on PET/CT scanner for radiotherapy planning with the aid of lasers.

Delineation of metabolic/structural target volumes

The advent of PET/CT planning has opened up new challenges in planning RT. There has been little guidance from the literature on how best to use PET/CT information in contouring tumor and target volumes and there are some new technical difficulties for the radiation oncologist to consider. Some types of PET information are easy to incorporate into treatment planning. A lymph node that is negative for tumor by CT criteria but is unequivocally involved on PET can easily be incorporated into the target volume. Changes to the perceived status of the thoracic lymph node stations have the biggest influence on changing target volumes in the treatment of NSCLC. Similarly, enlarged nodes that are not metabolically active on PET may be omitted from the GTV if considered unlikely to contain tumor, and this is simple to accomplish.

In contrast, there can be a major difficulty in determining the boundaries of some tumors that do not have clearly delineated margins on CT component of PET/CT [34]. This is due to the relatively low resolution of the PET part of the image and the consequent blurriness of the edge of many structures visualized on PET scans. When the edge of a tumor gradually merges into adjacent normal tissues, it can be difficult to decide where to place the contour that defines the edge of the lesion when determining the GTV. Motion of the patient on the couch top, which should be minimal with appropriate positioning and immobilization, and internal motion, such as that related to respiration or the cardiac cycle that can only be compensated

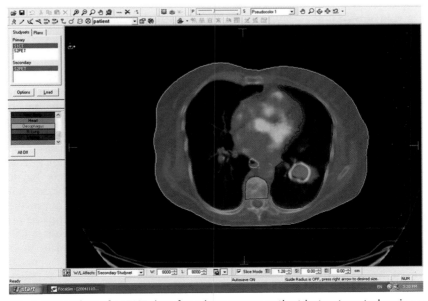

Fig. 3. Screenshot of PET/CT data for a lung cancer patient in treatment planning workstation.

for by gated acquisition of the PET data, also contribute to the blurriness of PET images. Other confounding factors may include regions of low avidity in the tumor due to necrosis and poor contrast between tumors with a low standardized uptake value and adjacent normal structures. Whereas CT information is acquired almost instantaneously and represents a snapshot in time, PET information is acquired over many respiratory and cardiac cycles and therefore represents an "average" position of the structures imaged. Tumor movement will be discussed further below.

There are two main approaches to contouring the edges of tumors on PET/CT. The first, which is preferred at our institution, is to use a standardized visual approach. At the Peter MacCallum Cancer Center (Melbourne, Australia), PET/CT data are displayed using uniform window settings and color settings. All available information is used in an "intelligent" process, including PET and CT data, biopsy reports, and the results of fluoroscopy to assess tumor movement. We have considerable institutional experience of comparing individual PET/CT scan information with surgical findings in operable cases and this experience is helpful in the planning process for unresectable tumors. The contouring of the GTV is only performed following consultation with the nuclear medicine physician who is asked to draw around the edge of the tumor on a hard copy of the PET/CT scan. Alternatively, the PET physician may be present in the radiotherapy planning area. Preliminary reproducibility studies at our center, so far unpublished, suggest that this approach gives similar results if the GTV is contoured by a radiologist, PET physician, or radiation oncologist. It must be emphasized that this approach should be used in the setting of a rigorous contouring protocol.

The second approach to contouring recognizes that visual methods can suffer from unacceptable variability due to human factors and makes use of the quantitative information available from PET. Various automated or semi-automated approaches are being tried for tumor contouring [32,35–37], but none of these methods has yet proven to be a comprehensive solution to the problem in vivo [38] although static phantoms can be effectively contoured [31]. In a clinical setting, all of the automated approaches must frequently be overridden by a human operator, because FDG uptake is not just due to malignant processes; it can also result from a range of inflammatory and physiological conditions that no computer software can recognize but often can be readily recognized by an experienced physician (eg, uptake in brown fat or muscle, sarcoidosis, and so forth). An increase in reproducibility could

potentially be associated with a decrease in accuracy unless each computer-derived tumor contour is carefully analyzed and edited by the radiation oncologist, who bears final responsibility for the planning process.

Movement

The region of three-dimensional space within which a lesion moves can be referred to as the internal target volume [31,37]. This is often well appreciated on PET scanning because of the long acquisition time. Metabolic lesions are usually qualitatively enlongated in the axes of respiratory movement compared with their true dimensions, reflecting temporal blurring of activity, unless the CT image is acquired using some form of gating. Because the lesion spends relatively less time at the extremes of respiratory excursion, particularly at the end of inspiration, activity tends to be less intense in those axial planes where the tumor spends proportionally less time. The PET-determined volume thus indicates most clearly the region of space where a tumor spends the most time. Accordingly a treatment centered on the PET-determined tumor volume is likely to be aimed correctly [39,40].

Role of PET in radiation therapy planning in non–small cell lung cancer

Lung cancer is the malignancy in which PET has had the greatest impact on selection of patients for radiotherapy and on radiotherapy planning [41]. This relates both to the clarity of imaging of a metabolically active cancer in a location favorable for PET and to the high rate of incremental abnormal findings seen on PET, compared with conventional imaging [42]. There is an abundance of evidence from surgical series, with systematic clinico-pathological correlation, proving that PET is much more accurate than CT in the assessment of thoracic lymph nodes, especially when CT and PET information are combined. Dwamena and colleagues [43] reviewed English-language reports on the performance of PET (14 studies, 514 patients) and CT (29 studies, 2226 patients). They reported that FDG-PET was significantly more accurate than CT ($P < .001$). The mean sensitivity was 0.79 for PET versus 0.60 for CT. The mean specificity was 0.91 for PET versus 0.77 for CT. These data can be extrapolated to radiotherapy candidates, for whom mediastinoscopy is not usually performed if the patient clearly has unresectable disease on the basis of CT findings or is medically unfit for surgery. Due to the expectation of a relatively high prevalence of nodal involvement in patients already selected for radiotherapy as the preferred treatment option, the positive predictive value of PET findings is likely to be even higher than that for surgical series, wherein a lower prevalence of mediastinal nodal involvement would tend to decrease the apparent positive predictive value allowing for a similar specificity of PET in both situations [44].

Another crucial advantage of PET is the ability to image distant metastases and thereby exclude patients who have incurable metastatic disease from futile aggressive attempts at cure [45]. In the absence of histopathology when imaging must be relied upon for radiotherapy planning, it is clear that the most reliable imaging for NSCLC, namely PET/CT, should be given the most weight in determining whom to treat and what anatomic sites to irradiate.

PET for selection of patients with non–small cell lung cancer for radical radiation therapy

In a large prospective study at the Peter MacCallum Cancer Centre, 153 patients who had NSCLC, all of whom were suitable candidates for radical RT on the basis of clinical assessment and conventional imaging, underwent PET scanning [11]. PET data were used for patient selection for radical RT and were also used to assist with RT planning in those who remained suitable. In that study, after PET, 30% of patients were considered unsuitable for radical RT because they had distant metastases (20%) or thoracic disease too extensive for radical irradiation (10%). Patients rejected for radical RT after PET were considered suitable only for palliative therapies and had very poor survival, but the remaining patients had very good results after aggressive therapy. A comparison of a prospective PET-staged cohort treated with radical RT/chemo RT with a comparable group of patients treated similarly in a phase III trial without PET staging at the same institution, showed that PET-staged patients had significantly better survival [28]. It is likely that this was primarily an effect of superior patient selection. Patients who had apparent stage III NSCLC, on the basis of non–PET staging investigations, had a significantly higher ($P = .016$) rate of detection of distant metastasis by PET (24%) than patients who had stage II (18%) or stage I disease (7.5%), a finding in keeping with Bayesian principles given that the ultimate distant failure rate is much higher in patients who have stage III disease [46]. The superior outcomes, however, could also have reflected superior treatment delivery in those deemed still suitable for treatment with curative intent.

Studies of PET in radiotherapy planning in lung cancer

NSCLC is the malignancy in which the effect of PET on RT planning has been most intensively studied and in which PET has had the greatest impact.

Despite this fact, knowledge in this area is still limited, and no convincing data have yet been published that demonstrate superior outcomes owing to incorporation of PET into RT planning beyond the effects of superior patient selection. Nevertheless, this is an area of intensive study, and all published studies indicate that target volumes determined using PET or PET/CT are often very different from those determined using CT alone. The greatest impact arises in patients for whom PET shows different lymph node status from CT, most commonly upstaging the extent of apparent nodal disease. A significant impact is also seen in patients who have atelectasis, where the boundary between tumor and collapsed/consolidated lung can only be identified with the aid of PET [47].

A number of studies have tried to quantify the impact of PET on RT planning in NSCLC. In our earliest study, we used PET rather than PET/CT and had no ability to coregister images [11]. Despite those limitations, we found that 22 of 102 patients had a significant increase in RT target volumes to cover new sites of disease seen only on PET. In 16 patients the target volume was reduced because regions of bland atelectasis could be excluded or enlarged nodes proved not to be FDG-avid. In 1998, Nestle and colleagues [47] reported that a significant increase in the radiation field was required to cover PET-detected disease in 9% of 34 patients, but a significant decrease was seen in 26%, especially those who had atelectasis. Munley and colleages [48] recorded that 35% of 35 patients had an increase in the RT field as a result of PET. In a larger study of 73 patients, Vanuytsel and colleagues [49] found that there was an increase in GTV in 22% of patients and a decrease in 40%. Other significant studies include work by Bradley and colleagues [50], who used coregistered sequential PET and CT scans and reported increased GTV in 46% and reduced GTV in 12%. Brianzoni and colleagues [51] reported that GTV/CTV was increased in 44% and reduced in 6% of 24 lung cancer patients planned using a dedicated PET/CT scanner. Fig. 4 illustrates the difference between a PTV obtained using CT alone and one obtained using PET/CT in a patient from our current prospective RT planning trial in NSCLC.

Studies that did not use dedicated PET scanners for treatment planning have not been considered here because we believe that the lower sensitivity of coincidence scanners, especially for small nodes, represents a significant disadvantage compared with true PET scanning in lung cancer. Because PET-based staging is much more accurate than CT-based staging and because numerous studies have shown that radiotherapy treatment fields are significantly different if PET is used, we recommend that

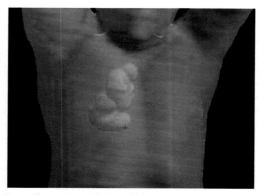

PET should be used in radiotherapy planning for NSCLC if it is available. Because of the very poor long-term locoregional disease control rates with RT in lung cancer [52], there is increasing interest in dose escalation of RT [53–56]. This could potentially lead to superior local control and survival but only if RT is appropriately directed. The authors believe that dose escalation without PET in many cases will be futile.

Role of PET in small cell lung cancer

Limited stage small cell lung cancer (SCLC) is potentially curable, with especially good results reported for patients treated using concurrent chemoradiation with twice daily RT fractionation. Patients who attain a complete response after primary or "induction" therapy for SCLC are at high risk for relapse with brain metastasis unless they receive prophylactic cranial irradiation. Extensive stage disease is generally considered to be incurable and is managed with chemotherapy alone. SCLC is well imaged by PET, but because it is less common than NSCLC and because treatment is often commenced soon after diagnosis because of its rapid growth rate, there are no large published series reporting the results of PET staging or restaging in this disease. At our own center, we reviewed 36 consecutive SCLC patients who underwent 47 PET studies for either staging (n = 11), restaging after therapy (n = 21), or both (n = 4). Of 15 patients who had PET for staging, 5 (33%) were upstaged-from limited to extensive disease and treated without thoracic radiotherapy [57]. Twenty-five patients underwent 32 restaging PET scans, of which 20 (63%) were discordant with conventional imaging. In 8 cases, PET showed more extensive disease than conventional imaging, and in 12 cases

PET-apparent disease appeared less extensive. In 13 patients, 14 untreated discordant lesions were evaluable; PET was confirmed accurate in 11 (79%) sites by last follow-up. These results are similar to those reported by other groups [58–62], suggesting that PET may have a role to play in selecting patients for RT and in designing the RT fields. PET may also be useful in defining complete remission more accurately so that patients may be appropriately selected for PCI.

Potential for new tracers

Although FDG provides an excellent combination of sensitivity and specificity for most clinical oncological settings, it should be recognized that it simply visualizes a basic biochemical function of most living cells (ie, their ability to use glucose as an energy substrate). Lack of specificity of glucose metabolism as a target for disease detection is particularly relevant for the detection of cancer. Because enhanced glycolytic metabolism is a characteristic of many cancers but also of active inflammatory processes, cancer staging can be compromised by apparent focal accumulations of FDG due to infectious diseases, granulomatous lesions, and inflammatory healing responses related to previous interventions or therapies. Although pattern recognition can play an important role in differentiating these processes [63], biopsy may be necessary to definitively confirm the nature of FDG PET abnormalities. Even when cancer is known to be present, high uptake in adjacent tissues due to physiologic processes can reduce lesion contrast and thereby impair the sensitivity of FDG-PET for the detection of disease. The most obvious example of this is in the brain where high glucose use by the normal cortex can mask the presence of brain tumors but can also happen in lung cancer where postobstructive pneumonia can impair differentiation of NSCLC from adjacent inflammatory changes. Low FDG avidity can also occur with certain tumors and reduce contrast and, therefore, sensitivity even in the absence of high background activity. Bronchioloalveolar lung cancer is but one example of tumors of this type [64]. New tracers offer the potential to address both these limitations and also to establish new applications for PET, particularly in target disease specific clinical applications.

In an era where molecular profiling is identifying specific and mechanistically important alterations in diseased cells, a logical progression of PET tracer development is to go beyond probing of basic biochemical processes to looking at more specific features of cancer biology. With respect to radiation oncology, the concept of subpopulations of cells with differing radiosensitivity and capacity for repopulation may be important to the design of treatment schedules and dose. Rapidly proliferating tumors may have greater potential for repopulation and thereby benefit from accelerated treatment regimens, as is exemplified by the results of continuous hyperfractuioinated accelerated radiotherapy (CHART) in NSCLC [65] or head and neck cancer [66]. Alternatively, hypoxic cells often have a low proliferative fraction and are more likely to be radioresistant. Both these processes can now be imaged with PET. The cellular uptake of fluorothymidine provides evaluation of cellular proliferation and has been found to correlate with the immunohistochemical proliferation marker ki-67 [67].

Extensive efforts have also been made to develop PET tracers to enable the noninvasive imaging of hypoxia. ^{18}F-fluoromisonidazole (FMISO) is the most extensively studied agent and has been shown to stratify prognosis in patients receiving conventional radiotherapy [27,68]. However, FMISO is a relatively lipophilic compound and demonstrates relatively low uptake in hypoxic tissue relative to normal tissue, and slow clearance from normal tissues requiring delayed scanning with consequences on contrast and image quality. This has led to the development of other hypoxic tracers with more favorable imaging properties. ^{18}F-fluoro-azomycin arabinoside (FAZA) is one such agent [69]. Preliminary results have been obtained at our institution with the use of FAZA to image hypoxia within head and neck squamous cell carcinomas. These suggest that FAZA is likely to be a superior agent for hypoxia imaging and it may have applicability in lung cancer.

^{18}F-fluoromethyl-dimethyl-2-hydroxyethyl-ammonium or fluorocholine (FCH) is also an interesting new tracer. Tumor tissues have a requirement for increased synthesis of phosphatidylcholine, an important constituent of cell membranes. Increased rates of transmembrane transport and subsequent phosphorylation of choline by the enzyme choline kinase in tumors have been demonstrated. Preliminary studies suggest that FCH may be more sensitive than FDG for detection of nodal and bone metastases in prostate cancer [70]. In defining the need and extent of radiotherapy for suspected nodal involvement in patients who have prostate cancer, FCH may prove superior to FDG because of higher sensitivity for disease detection.

Summary

PET is transforming the way radiation oncologists approach lung cancer and is contributing to increasing optimism in our approach to this group of diseases. PET has an even bigger impact on the management of patients who have lung cancer treated with radiation than on those managed with surgery. This is because of the very high rates of abnormal findings in patients who have more advanced disease and because RT candidates do not undergo comprehensive surgical staging. PET selection alone is enough to improve our apparent success rate with this modality. PET/CT therefore represents the best quality information that we can get for most patients, and it differs considerably from the information that we previously obtained from CT alone. The authors believe that we are in the early stages of a revolution in thoracic oncology, one in which PET staging will become a standard part of the evaluation of all patients who are candidates for definitive RT for lung cancer and in which PET data will be seamlessly integrated into the treatment planning process.

References

[1] Chang JY, Liu HH, Komaki R. Intensity modulated radiation therapy and proton radiotherapy for non-small cell lung cancer. Curr Oncol Rep 2005;7(4):255–9.

[2] Svensson H, Moller TR. Developments in radiotherapy. Acta Oncol 2003;42(5–6):430–42.

[3] Drzymala RE, Mohan R, Brewster L, et al. Dose-volume histograms. Int J Radiat Oncol Biol Phys 1991;21(1):71–8.

[4] Ling CC, Burman C, Chui CS, et al. Conformal radiation treatment of prostate cancer using inversely-planned intensity-modulated photon beams produced with dynamic multileaf collimation. Int J Radiat Oncol Biol Phys 1996; 35(4):721–30.

[5] Leibel SA, Fuks Z, Zelefsky MJ, et al. Intensity-modulated radiotherapy. Cancer J 2002;8(2): 164–76.

[6] Pickles T, Pollack A. The case for dose escalation versus adjuvant androgen deprivation therapy for intermediate risk prostate cancer. Can J Urol 2006;13(Suppl 2):68–71.

[7] Bussels B, Maes A, Hermans R, et al. Recurrences after conformal parotid-sparing radiotherapy for head and neck cancer. Radiother Oncol 2004; 72(2):119–27.

[8] Mountain CF. Lung cancer staging classification. Clin Chest Med 1993;14(1):43–53.

[9] Luciani A, Itti E, Rahmouni A, et al. Lymph node imaging: basic principles. Eur J Radiol 2006; 58(3):338–44.

[10] Webb WR, Gatsonis C, Zerhouni EA, et al. CT and MR imaging in staging non-small cell bronchogenic carcinoma: report of the Radiologic Diagnostic Oncology Group. Radiology 1991; 178(3):705–13.

[11] MacManus MP, Hicks RJ, Ball DL, et al. F-18 fluorodeoxyglucose positron emission tomography staging in radical radiotherapy candidates with

nonsmall cell lung carcinoma: powerful correlation with survival and high impact on treatment. Cancer 2001;92(4):886–95.

[12] Vansteenkiste JF, Stroobants SG. Positron emission tomography in the management of non-small cell lung cancer. Hematol Oncol Clin North Am 2004;18(1):269–88.

[13] Wirth A, Seymour JF, Hicks RJ, et al. Fluorine-18 fluorodeoxyglucose positron emission tomography, gallium-67 scintigraphy, and conventional staging for Hodgkin's disease and non-Hodgkin's lymphoma. Am J Med 2002; 112(4):262–8.

[14] Jerusalem G, Beguin Y, Fassotte MF, et al. Whole-body positron emission tomography using 18F-fluorodeoxyglucose for posttreatment evaluation in Hodgkin's disease and non-Hodgkin's lymphoma has higher diagnostic and prognostic value than classical computed tomography scan imaging. Blood 1999;94(2):429–33.

[15] Pramesh CS, Mistry RC. Role of PET scan in management of oesophageal cancer. Eur J Surg Oncol 2005;31(4):449.

[16] Flamen P, Lerut A, Van Cutsem E, et al. Utility of positron emission tomography for the staging of patients with potentially operable esophageal carcinoma. J Clin Oncol 2000;18(18): 3202–10.

[17] Grigsby PW, Siegel BA, Dehdashti F. Lymph node staging by positron emission tomography in patients with carcinoma of the cervix. J Clin Oncol 2001;19(17):3745–9.

[18] Follen M, Levenback CF, Iyer RB, et al. Imaging in cervical cancer. Cancer 2003;98(9 Suppl): 2028–38.

[19] Kalff V, Hicks RJ, Ware RE, et al. Evaluation of high-risk melanoma: comparison of [18F]FDG PET and high-dose 67Ga SPET. Eur J Nucl Med Mol Imaging 2002;29(4):506–15.

[20] Wagner JD. Fluorodeoxyglucose positron emission tomography for melanoma staging: refining the indications. Ann Surg Oncol 2006;13(4): 444–6.

[21] Hicks RJ, Toner GC, Choong PF. Clinical applications of molecular imaging in sarcoma evaluation. Cancer Imaging 2005;5(1):66–72.

[22] Esteves FP, Schuster DM, Halkar RK. Gastrointestinal tract malignancies and positron emission tomography: an overview. Semin Nucl Med 2006;36(2):169–81.

[23] Gyorke T, Zajic T, Lange A, et al. Impact of FDG PET for staging of Ewing sarcomas and primitive neuroectodermal tumours. Nucl Med Commun 2006;27(1):17–24.

[24] Franzius C, Schober O. Assessment of therapy response by FDG PET in pediatric patients. Q J Nucl Med 2003;47(1):41–5.

[25] Floeth FW, Pauleit D, Wittsack HJ, et al. Multimodal metabolic imaging of cerebral gliomas: positron emission tomography with [18F]fluoroethyl-L-tyrosine and magnetic resonance spectroscopy. J Neurosurg 2005;102(2):318–27.

[26] Yap CS, Czernin J, Fishbein MC, et al. Evaluation of thoracic tumors with 18F-fluorothymidine and 18F-fluorodeoxyglucose-positron emission tomography. Chest 2006;129(2):393–401.

[27] Rischin D, Hicks RJ, Fisher R, et al. Prognostic significance of [18F]-misonidazole positron emission tomography-detected tumor hypoxia in patients with advanced head and neck cancer randomly assigned to chemoradiation with or without tirapazamine: a substudy of Trans-Tasman Radiation Oncology Group Study 98.02. J Clin Oncol 2006;24(13):2098–104.

[28] MacManus MP, Wong K, Hicks RJ, et al. Early mortality after radical radiotherapy for non-small-cell lung cancer: comparison of PET-staged and conventionally staged cohorts treated at a large tertiary referral center. Int J Radiat Oncol Biol Phys 2002;52(2):351–61.

[29] Ling CC, Humm J, Larson S, et al. Towards multidimensional radiotherapy (MD-CRT): biological imaging and biological conformality. Int J Radiat Oncol Biol Phys 2000;47(3): 551–60.

[30] Austin-Seymour M, Kalet I, McDonald J, et al. Three dimensional planning target volumes: a model and a software tool. Int J Radiat Oncol Biol Phys 1995;33(5):1073–80.

[31] Caldwell CB, Mah K, Skinner M, et al. Can PET provide the 3D extent of tumor motion for individualized internal target volumes? A phantom study of the limitations of CT and the promise of PET. Int J Radiat Oncol Biol Phys 2003; 55(5):1381–93.

[32] Ciernik IF, Huser M, Burger C, et al. Automated functional image-guided radiation treatment planning for rectal cancer. Int J Radiat Oncol Biol Phys 2005;62(3):893–900.

[33] Ackerly T, Andrews J, Ball D, et al. Display of positron emission tomography with Cadplan. Australas Phys Eng Sci Med 2002;25(2):67–77.

[34] Nestle U, Kremp S, Schaefer-Schuler A, et al. Comparison of different methods for delineation of 18F-FDG PET-positive tissue for target volume definition in radiotherapy of patients with non-Small cell lung cancer. J Nucl Med 2005;46(8):1342–8.

[35] Davis JB, Reiner B, Huser M, et al. Assessment of (18)F PET signals for automatic target volume definition in radiotherapy treatment planning. Radiother Oncol 2006;80(1):43–50.

[36] Drever L, Robinson DM, McEwan A, et al. A local contrast based approach to threshold segmentation for PET target volume delineation. Med Phys 2006;33(6):1583–94.

[37] Chetty IJ, Fernando S, Kessler ML, et al. Monte Carlo-based lung cancer treatment planning incorporating PET-defined target volumes. J Appl Clin Med Phys 2005;6(4):65–76.

[38] Yaremko B, Riauka T, Robinson D, et al. Thresholding in PET images of static and moving targets. Phys Med Biol 2005;50(24): 5969–82.

[39] Steenbakkers RJ, Duppen JC, Fitton I, et al. Observer variation in target volume delineation of lung cancer related to radiation oncologist-computer interaction: a 'big brother' evaluation. Radiother Oncol 2005;77(2):182–90.

[40] Jin JY, Ajlouni M, Chen Q, et al. A technique of using gated-CT images to determine internal target volume (ITV) for fractionated stereotactic lung radiotherapy. Radiother Oncol 2006; 78(2):177–84.

[41] Mac Manus MP, Hicks RJ. PET scanning in lung cancer: current status and future directions. Semin Surg Oncol 2003;21(3):149–55.

[42] Gilman MD, Aquino SL. State-of-the-art FDG-PET imaging of lung cancer. Semin Roentgenol 2005;40(2):143–53.

[43] Dwamena BA, Sonnad SS, Angobaldo JO, et al. Metastases from non-small cell lung cancer: mediastinal staging in the 1990s–meta-analytic comparison of PET and CT. Radiology 1999; 213(2):530–6.

[44] Dendukuri N, Rahme E, Belisle P, et al. Bayesian sample size determination for prevalence and diagnostic test studies in the absence of a gold standard test. Biometrics 2004;60(2):388–97.

[45] MacManus MR, Hicks R, Fisher R, et al. FDG-PET-detected extracranial metastasis in patients with non-small cell lung cancer undergoing staging for surgery or radical radiotherapy–survival correlates with metastatic disease burden. Acta Oncol 2003;42(1):48–54.

[46] MacManus MP, Hicks RJ, Matthews JP, et al. High rate of detection of unsuspected distant metastases by pet in apparent stage III non-small-cell lung cancer: implications for radical radiation therapy. Int J Radiat Oncol Biol Phys 2001; 50(2):287–93.

[47] Nestle U, Walter K, Schmidt S, et al. 18F-deoxy-glucose positron emission tomography (FDG-PET) for the planning of radiotherapy in lung cancer: high impact in patients with atelectasis. Int J Radiat Oncol Biol Phys 1999;44(3):593–7.

[48] Munley MT, Marks LB, Scarfone C, et al. Multimodality nuclear medicine imaging in three-dimensional radiation treatment planning for lung cancer: challenges and prospects. Lung Cancer 1999;23(2):105–14.

[49] Vanuytsel LJ, Vansteenkiste JF, Stroobants SG, et al. The impact of (18)F-fluoro-2-deoxy-D-glucose positron emission tomography (FDG-PET) lymph node staging on the radiation treatment volumes in patients with non-small cell lung cancer. Radiother Oncol 2000;55(3):317–24.

[50] Bradley J, Thorstad WL, Mutic S, et al. Impact of FDG-PET on radiation therapy volume delineation in non-small-cell lung cancer. Int J Radiat Oncol Biol Phys 2004;59(1):78–86.

[51] Brianzoni E, Rossi G, Ancidei S, et al. Radiotherapy planning: PET/CT scanner performances in the definition of gross tumor volume and clinical target volume. Eur J Nucl Med Mol Imaging 2005;32(12):1392–9.

[52] Mac Manus MP, Hicks RJ, Matthews JP, et al. Metabolic (FDG-PET) response after radical radiotherapy/chemoradiotherapy for non-small cell lung cancer correlates with patterns of failure. Lung Cancer 2005;49(1):95–108.

[53] Chen M, Hayman JA, Ten Haken RK, et al. Long-term results of high-dose conformal radiotherapy for patients with medically inoperable T1–3N0 non-small-cell lung cancer: is low incidence of regional failure due to incidental nodal irradiation? Int J Radiat Oncol Biol Phys 2006;64(1):120–6.

[54] Nelson C, Starkschall G, Chang JY. The potential for dose escalation in lung cancer as a result of systematically reducing margins used to generate planning target volume. Int J Radiat Oncol Biol Phys 2006;65(2):573–86.

[55] Kong FM, Ten Haken RK, Schipper MJ, et al. High-dose radiation improved local tumor control and overall survival in patients with inoperable/unresectable non-small-cell lung cancer: long-term results of a radiation dose escalation study. Int J Radiat Oncol Biol Phys 2005;63(2):324–33.

[56] Chang DT, Zlotecki RA, Olivier KR. Re-examining the role of elective nodal irradiation: finding ways to maximize the therapeutic ratio. Am J Clin Oncol 2005;28(6):597–602.

[57] Blum R, MacManus MP, Rischin D, et al. Impact of positron emission tomography on the management of patients with small-cell lung cancer: preliminary experience. Am J Clin Oncol 2004; 27(2):164–71.

[58] Bradley JD, Dehdashti F, Mintun MA, et al. Positron emission tomography in limited-stage small-cell lung cancer: a prospective study. J Clin Oncol 2004;22(16):3248–54.

[59] Brink I, Schumacher T, Mix M, et al. Impact of [18F]FDG-PET on the primary staging of small-cell lung cancer. Eur J Nucl Med Mol Imaging 2004;31(12):1614–20.

[60] Pandit N, Gonen M, Krug L, et al. Prognostic value of [18F]FDG-PET imaging in small cell lung cancer. Eur J Nucl Med Mol Imaging 2003;30(1):78–84.

[61] Kamel EM, Zwahlen D, Wyss MT, et al. Whole-body (18)F-FDG PET improves the management of patients with small cell lung cancer. J Nucl Med 2003;44(12):1911–7.

[62] Chin R Jr, McCain TW, Miller AA, et al. Whole body FDG-PET for the evaluation and staging of small cell lung cancer: a preliminary study. Lung Cancer 2002;37(1):1–6.

[63] Hicks RJ, Mac Manus MP, Matthews JP, et al. Early FDG-PET imaging after radical radiotherapy for non-small-cell lung cancer: inflammatory changes in normal tissues correlate with tumor response and do not confound therapeutic response evaluation. Int J Radiat Oncol Biol Phys 2004;60(2):412–8.

[64] Heyneman LE, Patz EF. PET imaging in patients with bronchioloalveolar cell carcinoma. Lung Cancer 2002;38(3):261–6.

[65] Saunders M, Dische S, Barrett A, et al. Continuous hyperfractionated accelerated radiotherapy (CHART) versus conventional radiotherapy in non-small-cell lung cancer: a randomised multicentre trial. CHART Steering Committee. Lancet 1997;350(9072):161–5.

[66] Saunders MI, Dische S, Barrett A, et al. Randomised multicentre trials of CHART vs conventional radiotherapy in head and neck and non-small-cell lung cancer: an interim report. CHART Steering Committee. Br J Cancer 1996; 73(12):1455–62.

[67] Vesselle H, Grierson J, Muzi M, et al. In vivo validation of 3′deoxy-3′-[(18)F]fluorothymidine ([(18)F]FLT) as a proliferation imaging tracer in humans: correlation of [(18)F]FLT uptake by positron emission tomography with Ki-67 immunohistochemistry and flow cytometry in human lung tumors. Clin Cancer Res 2002; 8(11):3315–23.

[68] Eschmann SM, Paulsen F, Reimold M, et al. Prognostic impact of hypoxia imaging with 18F-misonidazole PET in non-small cell lung cancer and head and neck cancer before radiotherapy. J Nucl Med 2005;46(2):253–60.

[69] Piert M, Machulla HJ, Picchio M, et al. Hypoxia-specific tumor imaging with 18F-fluoroazomycin arabinoside. J Nucl Med 2005;46(1): 106–13.

[70] DeGrado TR, Coleman RE, Wang S, et al. Synthesis and evaluation of 18F-labeled choline as an oncologic tracer for positron emission tomography: initial findings in prostate cancer. Cancer Res 2001;61(1):110–7.

RADIOLOGIC
CLINICS
OF NORTH AMERICA

Radiol Clin N Am 45 (2007) 639–644

PET Versus PET/CT Dual-Modality Imaging in Evaluation of Lung Cancer

Lutz S. Freudenberg, MD, MA, MBA[a],*, Sandra J. Rosenbaum, MD[a],
Thomas Beyer, PhD[a], Andreas Bockisch, MD, PhD[a],
Gerald Antoch, MD[b]

- FDG-PET/CT versus FDG-PET
- FDG-PET/CT versus FDG-PET and CT read side by side
- Optimized PET/CT protocol

- *Breathing*
- *Contrast agents*
- Summary
- References

Lung cancer is the leading cause of tumor-related deaths [1]. Although rates of bronchial carcinoma–related death in men have decreased on average by 1.8% annually during the past decade, the incidence of lung cancer in women is increasing [1]. Non–small cell lung cancer (NSCLC) accounts for approximately 80% of bronchogenic malignancies. Among the 150 factors that help determine NSCLC prognosis, the tumor stage, as defined by the American Joint Committee on Cancer is considered to be the most important [2,3]. Thus, the choice of therapy options, including surgery, radiation therapy, and chemotherapy—used alone or in combination [4,5]—is based on the tumor stage. Consequently, the accurate determination of tumor size, potential infiltration of adjacent structures, mediastinal lymph node involvement, and the detection of distant metastases are of central importance. Especially the diagnosis of contralateral lymph node metastases and distant metastases is crucial (stage IIIB and stage V) as these exclude a curative therapeutic approach [6].

In general, morphological imaging with CT is the method of choice to define the extent of the primary tumor and to assess the tumor. However, one of the main limitations of CT is that it has a low accuracy when differentiating benign from malignant lymph nodes using a size criterion of 1 cm for mediastinal nodes and 7 mm for hilar nodes [7–9]. The limitations of this size-based node characterization system is well documented: up to 21% of nodes smaller than 10 mm are malignant, whereas 40% of nodes larger than 10 mm are benign [8–11].

In contrast, metabolic imaging using fluorine-18-2-fluoro-2-deoxy-D-glucose (FDG) positron emission tomography (PET) has been shown to be substantially more sensitive and specific in the detection and characterization of metastases to mediastinal lymph nodes (Fig. 1). Several studies compared the accuracy of CT and FDG-PET [6,11–14]: in a meta-analysis on staging lung cancer with PET and CT, Dwamena and colleagues [11] concluded that FDG-PET was significantly more accurate than CT and reported sensitivity and specificity

This article was previously published in PET Clinics 2006;1:347–52.
[a] Department of Nuclear Medicine, University of Duisburg, Hufelandstrasse 55 D-45122, Essen, Germany
[b] Department of Diagnostic and Interventional Radiology, University of Duisburg, Hufelandstrasse 55, D-45122 Essen, Germany
* Corresponding author.
E-mail address: lutz.freudenberg@uni-essen.de (L.S. Freudenberg).

doi:10.1016/j.rcl.2007.05.003

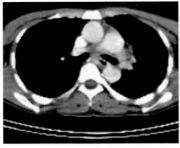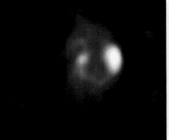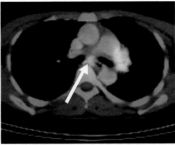

Fig. 1. CT (*left*), FDG-PET (*middle*), and FDG-PET/CT (*right*) of a 49-year-old male with diagnosis of NSCLC before neoadjuvant combined radiotherapy/chemotherapy. CT and FDG-PET clearly visualize a vital hilar metastasis. FDG-PET additionally shows additional tracer-uptake mediastinally. Exact localization is difficult due to little anatomic detail, CT alone is ambiguous. Integrated FDG-PET/CT allows diagnosis of a vital infracarinal metastasis (*arrow*).

values of 79% and 91% for PET and 60% and 77% for CT, respectively. Weber and colleagues [6], in a recent meta-analysis according to the Agency for Health Care Policy Research criteria, reported a significantly increased sensitivity and specificity of FDG-PET compared with CT in assessment of mediastinal lymph nodes and distant metastases with a sensitivity of 83% (95% CI: 75%–89%), and 96% (95% CI: 89%–99%), respectively. Based on FDG-PET findings, 18% of the patients received a different therapy compared with CT [6].

On the other hand, limited anatomic information in FDG-PET images frequently renders localization of a lesion and its potential infiltration into adjacent organs difficult [15,16]. Thus, for maximal diagnostic benefit, functional data sets should be read in conjunction with morphologic images. Image fusion and side-by-side image evaluation of morphologic and functional data sets have been proposed [17]. However, differences in patient positioning and motion-induced data misregistration cause image fusion of separately acquired CT and PET image sets to be complex and often unsatisfactory [18,19]. This limitation can be overcome by collecting functional and morphologic data in one examination. The availability of dual-modality PET/CT tomographs provides the technical basis for intrinsically aligned functional and morphologic data sets [19].

The purpose of this article is to summarize the accuracy of dual-modality FDG-PET/CT imaging in staging of NSCLC as compared with FDG-PET alone, and with FDG-PET as well as CT read side by side. Furthermore, an optimized PET/CT protocol for patients who have lung cancer is outlined.

FDG-PET/CT versus FDG-PET

Several studies have reported a higher sensitivity of FDG-PET/CT compared with FDG-PET alone.

For tumor staging, the sole use of conventional FDG-PET is limited based on the limited anatomical data. Thus, tumor size and a potential infiltration may be difficult to assess on PET alone. It has been shown in recent studies that in tumor staging of patients who have lung cancer, analysis of integrated FDG-PET/CT images is superior to that of FDG-PET or CT images alone when assessing the tumor stage [20–23]. The integration of morphologic CT and functional PET data sets particularly enables the most accurate differentiation of viable tumor tissue relative to all adjacent structures (eg, differentiation of tumor from atelectasis, detection of focal chest wall infiltration or mediastinal invasion) (**Fig. 2**) [20–22,24].

Furthermore, PET/CT resulted in further improvement of N staging compared with PET alone due to the ability to reveal the exact location of metastatic lymph nodes: accurate anatomic correlation is of benefit for exact localization of a solitary lymph node metastasis and thus allows exact classification as N1 or N2 disease, which is difficult but important [25]. Furthermore, FDG-PET/CT is important when identifying supraclavicular N3 disease (**Fig. 3**) [20,22,23,26]. Results of recent studies with respect to the tumor–node–metastasis

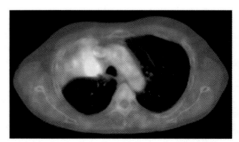

Fig. 2. FDG-PET/CT of a 47-year-old male with diagnosis of NSCLC before first treatment. Integrated FDG-PET/CT enables the most accurate differentiation of viable tumor tissue relative to atelectasis.

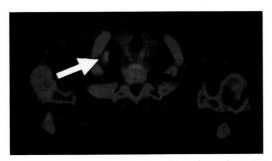

Fig. 3. FDG-PET/CT of a 54-year-old male with NSCLC (pancoast-tumor) showing a supraclavicular lymph node metastasis 0.5 cm in diameter not visible in CT alone and unambiguous in FDG-PET.

(TNM) system are summarized in Table 1. These studies reported significant advantages of FDG-PET/CT compared with FDG-PET alone.

It is generally concluded that dual-modality PET/CT represents the most efficient and accurate approach to NSCLC staging, with a profound effect on therapy and, hence, patient prognosis [20,22,23, 26,27]. Antoch and colleagues [26] described that PET/CT findings led to a change in tumor stage in 26% of patients compared with PET data alone, resulting in a change of treatment plans in 15%. Cerfolio and colleagues [20], Lardinois and colleagues [22], and Aquino and colleagues [23] likewise found tumor staging was significantly more accurate with integrated PET-CT than with PET alone, especially for stage I and stage II (see Table 1) [20,22,23,26,27].

In conclusion, dual-modality FDG-PET/CT data enabled more accurate staging of NSCLC than either FDG-PET or CT, reflecting the inherent limitations of these two imaging modalities when used alone. However, as Buell and colleagues [24]

argue, the somewhat unrealistic comparisons of FDG-PET alone with integrated FDG-PET/CT must show an advantage for FDG-PET/CT. To allow for a more balanced study design that reflects clinical reality, FDG-PET/CT must be compared with a side-by-side evaluation of conventional FDG-PET and CT scans.

FDG-PET/CT versus FDG-PET and CT read side by side

In general, visual correlation of CT and FDG-PET improves interpretation of both datasets [24,28]. For image coregistration, computer-assisted support appears helpful. However, in clinical practice, routine acceptance of retrospective image fusion may be limited by the complexity of retrospective coregistration algorithms and their limited accuracy for aligning areas of interest in independently acquired scans. Nonlinear registration techniques are required to account for complex patient motion, especially in the thorax and upper abdomen [29].

Several investigators have studied the impact of software image fusion in NSCLC showing significant improvement in staging of fused CT and FDG-PET data compared with FDG-PET alone [21,23, 24,30]. However, Vansteenkiste and colleagues [30] reported no significant differences between image fusion of FDG-PET and CT data compared with visual correlation. Halpern and colleagues [21] as well as Buell and colleagues [24] describe advantages of software fusion with regard to the T stage and the N stage when compared with FDG-PET alone.

Lardinois and colleagues [22] reported significant advantages of FDG-PET/CT over FDG-PET and CT read side by side when examining 50

Table 1: Sensitivity of FDG-PET versus FDG-PET/CT with respect to TNM and overall tumor staging (I–IV) according to American Joint Committee on Cancer

Study	Patients	TNM	FDG-PET	FDG-PET/CT	P value
Cerfolio et al [20]	129	T	38%–70%	50%–100%	.001
		N	60%–80%	77%–92%	.008
		M	81%–82%	90%–92%	NS
		Overall staging	17%–83%	50%–94%	NR
Halpern et al [21]	36	T	67%	97%	<.05
		Overall staging	57%	83%	<.05
Lardinois et al [22]	50	N	49%	93%	.013
		Overall staging	40%	88%	.001
Aquino et al [23]	45	N	59%–76%	71%–76%	.01
		Overall staging	53%–62%	73%–76%	.002
Antoch et al [26]	27	Overall staging	74%	96%	<.05
Shim et al [27]	106	N	–	85%	–
Keidar et al [31]	42	Restaging	96%	96%	NS

Abbreviations: NR, not reported; NS, not significant.

patients who have surgically staged NSCLC. They report a diagnostic accuracy for integrated FDG-PET/CT and visual correlation of FDG-PET and CT of 89% and 77%, respectively. This difference was statistically significant. Furthermore, they found additional information by FDG-PET/CT in 41% of their patients. However, as Buell and colleagues [24] note, this advantage of PET/CT was achieved by evaluating a multitude of different parameters, some of which were only of limited clinical relevance. Keidar and colleagues [31] performed a study addressing the diagnostic value of FDG-PET/CT versus FDG-PET and CT read side by side in suspected lung cancer recurrence showing no differences in sensitivity. Although FDG-PET/CT performed better with respect to specificity and positive predictive values, these results did not reach the level of statistical significance.

Two recent studies evaluated the accuracy of PET/CT and included oncology patients who have different malignancies. Their results are of interest with respect to NSCLC, because patients who have lung cancer represent the largest patient cohort within both patient populations. Antoch and colleagues [32] evaluated FDG-PET/CT for tumor staging in 260 patients who have solid tumors (57 patients who have NSCLC) and conclude that FDG-PET/CT is able to detect significantly more lesions than FDG-PET or CT alone. Based on a change in the TNM stage, they reported a change in patient management in 6% of patients who have FDG-PET/CT compared with FDG-PET and CT evaluated side by side. Buell and colleagues [24] evaluated side-by-side analysis of CT and conventional FDG-PET in 733 patients (174 who have bronchial cancer) with respect to patient groups that may benefit the most from the integrated PET/CT scanners. They showed that side-by-side reading of FDG-PET and CT failed to yield conclusive data with regard to lesion characterization in only 7.4% of patients so FDG-PET/CT might have been helpful in these cases.

Until now, only one study has evaluated the differences of integrated FDG-PET/CT versus software-based image fusion in NSCLC. Halpern and colleagues [21] reported equal results with regard to the T stage and the N stage for image fusion and PET/CT in cases in which software fusion was successful. However, software fusion of separately obtained PET and CT studies was successful in only 68% of the patients and failed in 32%. As stated by the authors, the performance of software fusion can significantly be improved when including transmission PET scans to a success rate from approximately 70% to 95% [33].

Further studies will have to evaluate the impact of integrated FDG-PET/CT versus software fusion keeping in mind that misregistration is not totally avoidable even with a combined PET/CT scanner [34,35]. Finally, the actual impact of more accurate tumor staging—beyond therapeutic decision making—on patient survival will have to be determined in future studies.

Optimized PET/CT protocol

Local misregistration between the CT and the PET in integrated PET/CT and the use of CT contrast media may bias the PET tracer distribution following CT-based attenuation correction [36]. Consequently, protocol requirements for PET/CT with diagnostic CT include alternative contrast application schemes to handle CT contrast agents appropriately. In addition, a special breathing protocol can avoid motion-induced artifacts in the area of the diaphragm. Using an optimized acquisition protocol significantly improves integrated PET/CT imaging and thus can further improve staging of NSCLC.

Breathing

The coregistration accuracy in combined PET/CT imaging is mainly impaired by respiration-induced mismatches between the CT and the PET. These artifacts are particularly severe when standard breath-hold techniques (eg, scanning at maximum inspiration) are transferred directly from clinical CT to combined PET/CT without further adaptation [34]. Goerres and colleagues [37] investigated the misregistration of pulmonary lesions with a combined PET/CT system and detected the mismatch between PET and CT to be most severe if the CT was performed during maximal inspiration of the patient. The registration error was found to be in the range of 5 to 33 mm in this setting [37,38]. Combined PET/CT scans during normal respiration go along with respiration artifacts in the majority of cases as well. To reduce potential misregistration from differences in the breathing pattern between two complementary PET and CT data sets, our protocol uses a limited breath-hold technique: patients are asked to hold their breath in normal expiration only for the time that the CT takes to cover the lower lung and liver, which is typically less than 15 seconds. Instructing the patient before the PET/CT examinations on the breath-hold command is essential in avoiding serious respiration artifacts [39]. When applying the limited breath-hold technique, the frequency of severe artifacts in the area of the diaphragm was reduced by half, and the spatial extent of respiration-induced artifacts can be reduced by at least 40% compared with the acquisition protocols without any breathing instructions [39].

With the introduction of multirow CT technology of up to 64 detector rows into PET/CT designs, the incidence of respiration artifacts in PET/CT examinations can further be reduced. This applies also to patients who are unable to follow any breath-hold instructions. For PET/CT imaging of normally breathing patients, a substantial improvement of image quality can be expected from employing CT technology with six or more detector rows as respiration-induced artifacts are reduced in both magnitude and prominence [38,40]. In conclusion, special breathing protocols are effective and should be used for CT scans as part of combined imaging protocols in dual-modality PET/CT.

Contrast agents

Standard application of intravenous CT contrast agents in combined PET/CT may lead to high-density artifacts on CT and attenuation-corrected PET [35]. To avoid associated diagnostic pitfalls, a special contrast injection protocol is needed. Comparing different protocols, Beyer and colleagues [41] found a reproducible high image quality in the CT image and in the attenuation-corrected PET image without high-density image artifacts when using a dual-phase injection (80 and 60 mL at 3 and 1.5 mL/s, respectively) of contrast agent in the caudocranial direction with a 50-second delay.

Summary

Software coregistration of FDG-PET and CT datasets as well as integrated FDG-PET/CT enable significantly more accurate assessment of NSCLC staging than either modality alone. Integrated FDG-PET/CT has been shown to be more accurate in NSCLC staging than FDG-PET and CT read side by side. However, the benefits of anatometabolic imaging using FDG-PET/CT can only be fully exploited if optimized acquisition protocols are implemented.

References

[1] Jemal A, Thomas A, Murray T, et al. Cancer statistics, 2002. CA Cancer J Clin 2002;52:23–47.

[2] Brundage MD, Davies D, Mackillop WJ. Prognostic factors in non-small cell lung cancer: a decade of progress. Chest 2002;122:1037–57.

[3] Greene FL, Page DL, Fleming ID, et al. AJCC cancer staging manual. 6th edition. New York: Springer; 2002.

[4] Smythe WR. Treatment of stage I and II non-small cell lung cancer. Cancer Control 2001;8: 318–25.

[5] Haura EB. Treatment of advanced nonsmall cell lung cancer: a review of current randomised clinical trials and an examination of emerging therapies. Cancer Control 2001;8:326–36.

[6] Weber WA, Dietlein M, Hellwig D, et al. PET with (18)F-fluorodeoxyglucose for staging of non-small cell lung cancer. Nuklearmedizin 2003;42: 135–44.

[7] Glazer GM, Gross BH, Quint LE, et al. Normal mediastinal lymph nodes: number and size according to American Thoracic Society mapping. AJR Am J Roentgenol 1985;144:261–5.

[8] Lowe VJ, DeLong DM, Hoffman JM, et al. Optimum scanning protocol for FDGPET evaluation of pulmonary malignancy. J Nucl Med 1995;36: 883–7.

[9] Deslauriers J, Gregoire J. Clinical and surgical staging of non-small cell lung cancer. Chest 2000;117:96S–103S.

[10] Staples CA, Muller NL, Miller RR, et al. Mediastinal nodes in bronchogenic carcinoma: comparison between CT and mediastinoscopy. Radiology 1988;167:367–72.

[11] Dwamena BA, Sonnad SS, Angobaldo JO, et al. Metastases from non-small cell lung cancer: mediastinal staging in the 1990s–meta-analytic comparison of PET and CT. Radiology 1999; 213:530–6.

[12] Adams S, Baum RP, Stuckensen T, et al. Prospective comparison of 18F-FDG PET with conventional imaging modalities (CT, MRI, US) in lymph node staging of head and neck cancer. Eur J Nucl Med 1998;25:1255–60.

[13] Marom EM, McAdams HP, Erasmus JJ, et al. Staging non-small cell lung cancer with whole-body PET. Radiology 1999;212:803–9.

[14] van Tinteren H, Hoekstra OS, Smit EF, et al. Effectiveness of positron emission tomography in the preoperative assessment of patients with suspected non-small-cell lung cancer: the PLUS multicentre randomised trial. Lancet 2002;359: 1388–93.

[15] Diederichs CG, Staib L, Vogel J, et al. Values and limitations of 18F-fluorodeoxyglucosepositron-emission tomography with preoperative evaluation of patients with pancreatic masses. Pancreas 2000;20:109–16.

[16] Weber WA, Avril N, Schwaiger M. Relevance of positron emission tomography (PET) in oncology. Strahlenther Onkol 1999;175:356–73.

[17] Wahl RL, Quint LE, Cieslak RD, et al. "Anatometabolic" tumor imaging: fusion of FDG PET with CT or MRI to localize foci of increased activity. J Nucl Med 1993;34:1190–7.

[18] Townsend DW. A combined PET/CT scanner: the choices. J Nucl Med 2001;42:533–4.

[19] Beyer T, Townsend DW, Blodgett TM. Dual-modality PET/CT tomography for clinical oncology. Q J Nucl Med 2002;46:24–34.

[20] Cerfolio RJ, Ojha B, Bryant AS, et al. The accuracy of integrated PET-CT compared with dedicated PET alone for the staging of patients with nonsmall cell lung cancer. Ann Thorac Surg 2004;78:1017–23.

[21] Halpern BS, Schiepers C, Weber WA, et al. Presurgical staging of non-small cell lung cancer:

positron emission tomography, integrated positron emission tomography/CT, and software image fusion. Chest 2005;128:2289–97.

[22] Lardinois D, Weder W, Hany TF, et al. Staging of non-small-cell lung cancer with integrated positron-emission tomography and computed tomography. N Engl J Med 2003;19:2500–7.

[23] Aquino SL, Asmuth JC, Alpert NM, et al. Improved radiologic staging of lung cancer with 2-[18F]-fluoro-2-deoxy-D-glucose-positron emission tomography and computed tomography registration. J Comput Assist Tomogr 2003;27:479–84.

[24] Buell U, Wieres FJ, Schneider W, et al. 18FDG-PET in 733 consecutive patients with or without side-by-side CT evaluation: analysis of 921 lesions. Nuklearmedizin 2004;43:210–6.

[25] Asamura H, Suzuki K, Kondo H, et al. Where is the boundary between N1 and N2 stations in lung cancer? Ann Thorac Surg 2000;70:1839–45.

[26] Antoch G, Stattaus J, Nemat AT, et al. Non-small cell lung cancer: dual-modality PET/CT in preoperative staging. Radiology 2003;229:526–33.

[27] Shim SS, Lee KS, Kim BT, et al. Non-small cell lung cancer: prospective comparison of integrated FDG PET/CT and CT alone for preoperative staging. Radiology 2005;236:1011–9.

[28] Reinartz P, Wieres FJ, Schneider W, et al. Side-by-side reading of PET and CT scans in oncology: which patients might profit from integrated PET/CT? Eur J Nucl Med Mol Imaging 2004;31:1456–61.

[29] Hutton BF, Braun M. Software for image registration: algorithms, accuracy, efficacy. Sem Nucl Med 2003;33:180–92.

[30] Vansteenkiste JF, Stroobants SG, Dupont PJ, et al. FDG-PET scan in potentially operable non-small cell lung cancer: do anatometabolic PET-CT fusion images improve the localisation of regional lymph node metastases? The Leuven Lung Cancer Group. Eur J Nucl Med 1998;25:1495–501.

[31] Keidar Z, Haim N, Guralnik L, et al. PET/CT using 18F-FDG in suspected lung cancer recurrence:

diagnostic value and impact on patient management. J Nucl Med 2004;45:1640–6.

[32] Antoch G, Saoudi N, Kuehl H, et al. Accuracy of whole-body dual-modality fluorine-18–2-fluoro-2-deoxy-D-glucose positron emission tomography and computed tomography (FDG-PET/CT) for tumor staging in solid tumors: comparison with CT and PET. J Clin Oncol 2004;22:4357–68.

[33] Slomka PJ, Dey D, Przetak C, et al. Automated 3-dimensional registration of stand-alone (18)F-FDG whole-body PET with CT. J Nucl Med 2003;44:1156–67.

[34] Beyer T, Antoch G, Muller S, et al. Acquisition protocol considerations for combined PET/CT imaging. J Nucl Med 2004;45(Suppl 1):25S–35S.

[35] Cohade C, Osman M, Marshall LN, et al. PET-CT: accuracy of PET and CT spatial registration of lung lesions. Eur J Nucl Med Mol Imaging 2003;30:721–6.

[36] Antoch G, Freudenberg LS, Egelhof T, et al. Focal tracer uptake: a potential artifact in contrast-enhanced dual-modality PET/CT scans. J Nucl Med 2002;43:1339–42.

[37] Goerres GW, Burger C, Schwitter MR, et al. PET/CT of the abdomen: optimizing the patient breathing pattern. Eur Radiol 2003;13:734–9.

[38] Goerres GW, Kamel E, Heidelberg TN, et al. PET/CT image co-registration in the thorax: influence of respiration. Eur J Nucl Med Mol Imaging 2002;29:351–60.

[39] Beyer T, Antoch G, Blodgett T, et al. Dual-modality PET/CT imaging: the effect of respiratory motion on combined image quality in clinical oncology. Eur J Nucl Med Mol Imaging 2003;30:588–96.

[40] Beyer T, Rosenbaum S, Veit P, et al. Respiration artifacts in whole-body (18)F-FDG PET/CT studies with combined PET/CT tomographs employing spiral CT technology with 1 to 16 detector rows. Eur J Nucl Med Mol Imaging 2005;32:1429–39.

[41] Beyer T, Antoch G, Bockisch A, et al. Optimized intravenous contrast administration for diagnostic whole-body 18F-FDG PET/CT. J Nucl Med 2005;46:429–35.

ELSEVIER
SAUNDERS

RADIOLOGIC
CLINICS
OF NORTH AMERICA

Radiol Clin N Am 45 (2007) 645–657

F-18 Fluorodeoxyglucose-Positron Emission Tomography Imaging for Primary Breast Cancer and Loco-Regional Staging

Norbert Avril, MD[a],*, Lee P. Adler, MD[b]

- Detection of primary breast tumors
- Positron emission tomography imaging
  of breast cancer
  *Positron emission tomography imaging
  procedure and image analysis
  in the breast*
  *Positron emission tomography imaging
  of the breast*

- *Biological features of breast cancer*
- Loco-regional staging
- Positron emission mammography
- Current clinical status of F-18
  fluorodeoxyglucose-positron emission
  tomography in primary breast cancer
- References

Breast cancer is the most common female malignancy in most European countries, North America, and Australia; it is less frequent in Asia and in Africa. In Europe, one out of every 10 to 15 women will develop breast cancer in her lifetime, and the risk is even higher in the United States, where it is one out of every eight women. Approximately 95% of breast cancer cases occur sporadically without any known genetic mutation, and the causal mechanisms underlying this disease have yet to be fully elucidated. Overall, 5-year survival rates are approximately 75%, with ranges of 92% for Stage I (pT1, pN0, M0) to 15% for Stage IV (M1) disease [1].

The main prognostic factors in patients who have breast cancer are lymph node status, tumor size, histologic grade, and the presence or absence of distant metastases. Most patients who have locally advanced disease have axillary lymph nodes involved

with their tumors, but a subset of patients have large primary tumors without lymph node involvement. For patients who have lymph node metastases, more than four lymph nodes involved predict poorer survival [2]. The College of American Pathologists has recently considered prognostic and predictive factors in breast cancer and stratified them into categories reflecting the strength of published evidence [3]. Factors ranked in Category I included tumor, node, metastases (TNM) staging; histologic grade; histologic type; mitotic figure counts; and hormone receptor status. Category II factors included c-erbB-2 (Her2-neu), proliferation markers, lymphatic and vascular channel invasion, and p53. Factors in Category III included DNA ploidy analysis, microvessel density, epidermal growth factor receptor, transforming growth factor-alpha, bcl-2, pS2, and cathepsin D.

This article was previously published in PET Clinics 2006;1:1–14.
[a] Department of Nuclear Medicine, Barts and the London School of Medicine, Queen Mary, University of London, West Smithfield (QEII), London, EC1A 7BE, UK
[b] Adler Institute for Advanced Imaging, The Pavilion, 261 Old York Road, Jenkintown, PA 19046, USA
* Corresponding author.
E-mail address: AvrilNE@upmc.edu (N. Avril).

doi:10.1016/j.rcl.2007.05.004

Invasive ductal carcinoma is the most common histological type (70%–80%), followed by invasive lobular carcinoma (6%–10%) and medullary carcinoma (∼ 3%). The remaining tumors include a variety of histological types. Invasive breast cancer may be present as a single tumor, or as multifocal if tumors are growing in the same quadrant of the breast, and as multicentric if they are detected in different quadrants. The disease can occur in any part of the breast, but most frequently occurs in the upper outer quadrant. Locally advanced breast cancer remains a particular challenge, because the majority of patients who have this diagnosis develop distant metastases despite appropriate therapy. Patients who have locally advanced disease include primary tumors with direct extension to chest wall or skin (stage T4); advanced nodal disease, such as fixed axillary nodes or involvement of ipsilateral supraclavicular, infraclavicular, or internal mammary nodes; and inflammatory carcinomas.

Noninvasive breast cancer consists of two histological and clinical subtypes: ductal and lobular in-situ carcinomas. The carcinoma cells are confined within the terminal duct lobular unit and the adjacent ducts, but have not yet invaded through the basement membrane. Generally, lobular carcinoma in situ (LCIS) does not present as a palpable tumor and is usually found incidentally in breast biopsies, often multifocal and bilateral. Ductal carcinoma in situ (DCIS) is increasingly diagnosed because of microcalcifications seen on mammograms, and is more likely to be confined to one breast or even to one quadrant of the breast.

If breast cancer is suspected, a biopsy is necessary to confirm the diagnosis. The National Comprehensive Cancer Network has published guidelines for the work-up of women who have newly diagnosed breast cancer. The recommendations include history and physical examination, diagnostic bilateral mammogram and ultrasound and optional breast MRI, pathology review, and determination of estrogen receptor, progesterone receptor, nuclear grade and HER-2/neu status. To evaluate distant metastases, chest radiograph, ultrasound of the abdomen, bone scintigraphy, and CT or MRI may be indicated.

Detection of primary breast tumors

Improved methods to detect and diagnose breast cancer early are required to achieve a significant impact on morbidity and mortality. More than 80% of cancers are detected because of a suspicious mass, either by self-examination or routine breast examination. Clinical signs include a fixed, hard mass; asymmetry of the breast contour; a protrusion; a subtle dimpling of the skin (peau d' orange); or a bloody nipple discharge. Depending on the size of the breast and the density of breast tissue, most tumors are not palpable smaller than 1 cm in diameter. Breast carcinomas are often present as irregularly shaped, firm or hard, yet painless nodules or masses. Physical examination typically does not allow an accurate differentiation between a malignant and a nonmalignant mass. Therefore, imaging modalities are used to improve the diagnostic accuracy, and various new and innovative technologies are being investigated for advancing the early detection and diagnosis of breast cancer.

Screening-mammography allows the detection of breast cancer earlier than breast self-examination, and is generally credited with earlier diagnosis and an overall improvement in survival for patients who have newly diagnosed breast cancer. Mammography localizes and assesses the extent of a lesion as well as identifying other suspicious masses. Studies in large series have shown that mammography, using mediolateral oblique and craniocaudal projections, is a useful tool to improve early detection of breast cancer. Depending on the lesion size and the radiographic appearance and breast tissue density, sensitivity ranges from 54% to 58% in women under age 40, and from 81% to 94% in those over 50 [4,5]. Malignant and benign breast lesions often display similar radiographic appearance, resulting in a major limitation of mammography [6]. A Breast Imaging Reporting and Data System (BI-RADS) has recently been introduced to characterize mammography [7]. The categories are listed and explained in Box 1.

In some studies, approximately 6 to 8 out of 10 patients who have suspicious lesions in mammography and who undergo surgery have benign histology [6,8]. A recent multicenter analysis of 332,926 diagnostic mammography examinations [9] found the positive predictive value of a biopsy recommendation to be 31.5%, and that of a biopsy performed

---

Box 1:   BI-RADS categories and definitions

0: More information is needed to give a final mammogram report.
1: Mammogram is normal.
2: Mammogram shows benign finding.
3: Probably benign finding—short interval follow-up suggested.
4: Suspicious abnormality—biopsy should be considered.
5: Highly suggestive of malignancy—appropriate action should be taken.

to be 39.5% This means that currently almost two thirds have a negative biopsy. For screening mammography, the positive predictive value is even lower. About 10% of breast carcinomas are not identified in mammography, even when they are palpable [10]. One reason is that mammography is limited, because cancer can have photon absorption similar to that of normal breast tissue, especially in younger women who have radiographically dense breasts. Despite these limitations, mammography is viewed as the best tool currently available for screening and early diagnosis.

Ultrasound has become an important imaging modality in evaluating the breast [11]. Ultrasound is often used in addition to mammography, and provides differentiation between cystic lesions and solid tumors. In younger patients who have dense breasts, ultrasound can be superior in the detection of breast cancer in comparison with mammography. Breast cancer typically shows irregularly shaped hypoechoic masses, posterior acoustical shadowing, and ill-defined demarcation against the surrounding tissue. Doppler ultrasound may help distinguish benign from malignant breast disease; however, the diagnostic accuracy is often not sufficient enough to accurately characterize abnormal tissue, and to specifically exclude malignancy [12]. Another common application of ultrasound is to provide guidance for interventional procedures [12,13]. Less common uses include assisting in staging of breast cancer and evaluating patients who have implants. Recently, there has been an interest in using ultrasound to screen asymptomatic women for breast cancer, as is done with mammography. Further studies must be performed to assess if this reduces mortality from breast cancer. Although primarily used to image the female breast, ultrasound also can be used to evaluate breast-related concerns in men. Uses of contrast-enhanced ultrasound are still experimental and would add an invasive component to an otherwise noninvasive study.

MRI has become a valuable tool in breast disease, especially in cases that are difficult to diagnose. Recent progress in both spatial and temporal resolutions, the imaging sequences used, pharmacokinetic modeling of contrast uptake, and the use of dedicated breast coils has contributed to the advancement of this imaging technique. More recently, phased-array breast coils, pulse sequences engineered to saturate signal from fat-containing tissue (FATSAT), and gadolinium-based contrast agents have done so as well [14]. MRI has several distinct advantages for breast imaging. These include three-dimensional visualization of breast tissue, information about tissue vascularity, and chest wall visualization. Moreover, MRI allows evaluation of dense breast parenchyma that often limits the detection of breast cancer in mammography. The use of paramagnetic contrast agents has been found to be essential in characterizing breast masses. Signal enhancement following injection of intravenous (IV) contrast is a highly sensitive criterion to detect breast cancer, and sensitivity is more than 90% in most studies. Unfortunately, the high sensitivity of MRI for invasive breast carcinomas is coupled with a correspondingly low specificity [14,15]. To improve upon the disappointingly low positive predictive value of enhancing lesions on MRI, high-speed dynamic imaging of the breast must be performed in make use of the differential washout rates of contrast agent gadolinium (III)-diethyltriaminepentaacetic acid (Gd-DTPA) in benign and malignant breast lesions. Even with dynamic imaging, MRI has not proven to be a robust technique for discriminating benign from malignant tumors in the community setting. MRI of the breast offers higher sensitivity for the detection of multifocal or multicentric cancer, which is important in selecting patients appropriate for breast-conserving surgery. It is also a valuable tool for the screening of patients who have a high risk of breast cancer, or in whom there is axillary disease or nipple discharge and conventional imaging has not revealed the primary focus. Lesions detected on MRI are frequently visible on mammography or ultrasound in retrospect, if not prospectively, allowing for subsequent biopsy. Techniques are also now available to biopsy lesions only apparent on MRI of the breast. MRI can differentiate scar tissue from tumor, and is specifically useful in patients suspected for local recurrent disease. Studies suggest that MRI can identify responders and nonresponders to neoadjuvant chemotherapy with more accuracy [16]. It is the modality of choice for the assessment of breast implants for rupture, with accuracy higher than radiograph mammography and ultrasound. The most important limitations of MRI beside the low specificity are patient compliance, scan time, and cost.

Positron emission tomography imaging of breast cancer

Positron emission tomography (PET) is a noninvasive imaging technique that measures the concentration of positron-emitting radiopharmaceuticals within the body. Depending upon the radiolabeled tracer used, PET can be used to determine various physiological and biochemical processes in vivo. PET is highly sensitive, with the capacity to detect picomolar concentrations of radiotracer, and provides superior image resolution compared with conventional nuclear medicine imaging with gamma cameras. Currently, PET imaging can target several biological features of cancer, including glucose metabolism, cell proliferation, perfusion, and hypoxia. Approximately 95% of clinical PET examinations are performed in patients who have known or suspected cancer, and virtually all of these are performed with a single radiotracer, the radiolabeled glucose analog, [F-18] 2-deoxy-2-fluoro-D-glucose (FDG). Following malignant transformation, various tumors are characterized by elevated glucose consumption and subsequent increased uptake and accumulation of FDG. PET imaging using FDG provides more sensitive and more specific information about the extent of disease than morphological/anatomical imaging alone. FDG-PET has become a standard imaging procedure for staging and restaging of many types of cancer [17]. In the United States, PET scans performed on patients who have head and neck cancer, follicular thyroid cancer, solitary pulmonary nodules, lung cancer, breast cancer, esophageal cancer, colorectal cancer, lymphoma, melanoma, and cervical cancer are generally considered reimbursable by third-party payers. The metabolic activity of neoplastic tissue assessed by PET offers additional information about cancer biology, and can be used for the differentiation between benign and malignant lesions, identification of early disease and staging of metastases, assessment of therapeutic effectiveness, and to determine tumor aggressiveness. The uptake mechanism and biochemical pathway of the glucose analog FDG has been extensively studied both in vitro and in vivo. The transport of the radiotracer through the cell membrane via glucose transport proteins, particularly glucose transporter type 1 (GLUT-1), and subsequent intracellular phosphorylation by hexokinase (HK) have been identified as key steps for subsequent tissue accumulation [18]. Because FDG-6-phosphate is not a suitable substrate for glucose-6-phosphate isomerase, and the enzyme level of glucose-6-phosphatase is generally low in tumors, FDG-6-phosphate accumulates in cells and is visualized by PET.

Positron emission tomography imaging procedure and image analysis in the breast

To ensure a standardized metabolic state, including low plasma glucose levels, oncology patients must fast for at least 4 to 6 hours before administration of FDG. Blood glucose level before tracer injection should ideally not exceed 150 mg/100 ml. Intravenous administration of about 300 to 400 MBq (∼10 mCi) F-18 FDG is used in most studies; however, Adler and colleagues [19,20] reported on a higher breast cancer detection rate using up to 750 MBq (∼20 mCi) F-18 FDG. To avoid artificial tracer retention in the axilla region, the tracer should be injected into an arm vein contralateral

to the suspected tumor. Most of the studies reported in literature are done in two-dimensional mode data acquisition, and the influence of three-dimensional mode on the results of breast imaging still needs to be studied. Imaging in prone position with both arms at the side and the breast hanging free is recommended to avoid compression and deformation of the breast. Data acquisition should be started approximately 60 minutes after tracer injection. Boerner and colleagues [21] showed increasing target-to-background ratios over time, suggesting a benefit to longer waiting periods between tracer injection and data acquisition. Lower image quality, due to radionuclide decay, has to be taken into account, however. Attenuation correction is recommended for optimal tumor localization as well as subsequent quantification of regional tracer uptake. The use of iterative reconstruction algorithms results in better image quality; an increase in diagnostic accuracy has not yet been reported. Visual image interpretation should include analysis of transaxial, coronal, and sagittal views. Breast cancer is typically present with focally increased FDG uptake, whereas benign tumors are negative in PET imaging. Proliferative mammary dysplasia may result in moderate but diffuse increased tracer uptake.

Attenuation-corrected PET images provide quantitative information about the tracer concentration in tissue. Various approaches of different complexity can be applied for quantitative PET analysis. Standardized uptake values (SUV) are frequently being calculated, providing a semiquantitative measure of FDG accumulation in tissue by normalizing the tissue radioactivity concentration measured with PET to injected dose and patient's body weight. Quantitative methods may be used to complement visual image analysis for differentiation between benign and malignant breast tumors; that is, by using an SUV-normalized scale for image display [22]. In particular, SUV correction for partial volume effects and normalization to blood glucose has been shown to yield the highest diagnostic accuracy for breast imaging. Corresponding threshold values for optimal tumor characterization have been published for various quantification methods [22]. Dynamic data acquisition allows calculation of the tracer influx constant, although this procedure is more complex and did not increase diagnostic accuracy.

Whole-body imaging can be improved by intravenous injection of furosemide (20–40 mg) to reduce tracer retention in the urinary system and butylscopolamine (20–40 mg) to reduce FDG uptake in the bowel [23]. Image evaluation requires an appreciation of the normal physiologic FDG uptake distribution and of variation between individuals, as well as consideration of artifacts and benign conditions that can mimic malignancy. Increased FDG uptake is found within the brain cortex, the myocardium, and the urinary tract. Low-to-moderate uptake is seen in the base of the tongue, salivary glands, thyroid, liver, spleen, gastrointestinal tract, bone marrow, musculature, and reproductive organs. Of particular importance is the inconsistent amount of normal uptake in glandular breast tissue. The most common normal cause of misinterpretation is related to muscle activity. Muscle tension may lead to increased FDG uptake, and physical activity immediately before or after tracer injection can lead to spurious muscle activity. In some patients, supraclavicular uptake has been shown to represent brown fat. Inflammatory and infectious processes also demonstrate increased FDG uptake, as well as some benign diseases, such as Paget's disease, Graves' disease, granulomatous disorders, healing fractures, and postradiation changes.

Positron emission tomography imaging of the breast

The first FDG imaging in breast cancer patients, using a collimated gamma camera, was reported in 1989 by Minn and Soini [24]. Shortly afterwards, Kubota and coworkers [25] reported on PET imaging with FDG in one case with local recurrence. In a first series of 10 patients who had locally advanced breast cancer, Wahl and colleagues [26] successfully identified all breast carcinomas. Subsequent studies including a limited number of patients, predominantly having advanced stages of disease, suggested a high accuracy of FDG-PET for the detection of primary breast carcinomas [Figs. 1–7] [19,24–26]. The largest patient group reported to date includes 144 patients who had 185 histologically confirmed breast tumors [27]. PET detected breast cancer with an overall sensitivity of 64.4% by conservative image reading (regarding only definite FDG uptake as positive), and 80.3% by sensitive image reading (regarding equivocal as well as definite FDG uptake as positive). When applying sensitive image reading, however, specificity decreased from 94.3% to 75.5% [27,28].

Schirrmeister and coworkers [29] found similar results in 117 patients, with a sensitivity of 93% and specificity of 75%. The use of non-attenuation-corrected PET imaging combined with sensitive imaging reading may have contributed to the higher sensitivity and lower specificity in this study. A recent study compared MR imaging of the breast with FDG-PET [30] found a comparable diagnostic accuracy (88% versus 84%) for both methods in 32 patients. The sensitivity of FDG-PET was 79%, whereas MRI detected all primary breast carcinomas; however, the specificity of FDG-PET was higher (94% versus 72%). Baslaim and coworkers [31] evaluated the usefulness of FDG-PET for diagnosing and staging

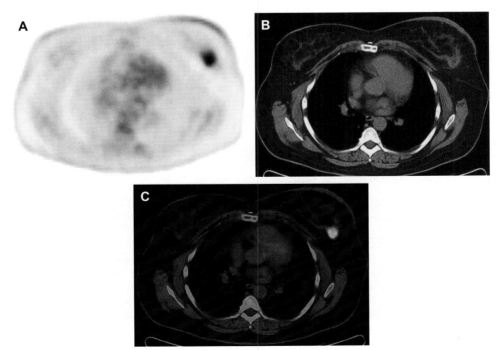

Fig. 1. Transaxial FDG-PET image (*A*), CT image (*B*), and fused PET/CT image (*C*), demonstrating a focal area of intense FDG uptake in the left breast.

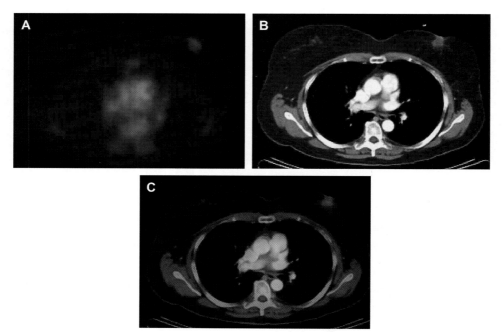

Fig. 2. Moderate FDG uptake in a local recurrence in the left breast. Transaxial FDG-PET (*A*), CT (*B*), and fused PET/CT (*C*).

of inflammatory breast cancer. All 7 patients studied presented with diffuse breast enlargement, redness, and peau d'orange. PET showed diffuse FDG uptake in the involved breast, with intense uptake in the primary tumor as well as increased FDG uptake in the skin.

The ability of PET to detect breast cancer greatly depends on tumor size. Regarding small tumors,

only 30 (68.2%) out of 44 breast carcinomas at stage pT1 (<2 cm) were correctly identified, compared with 57 (91.9%) out of 62 at stage pT2 (>2–5 cm) [27]. Sensitivity for tumors less than 1 cm (pT1a and b) was only 25%, compared with 84.4% for tumors between 1 and 2 cm in diameter (pT1c). Table 1 provides more detailed information.

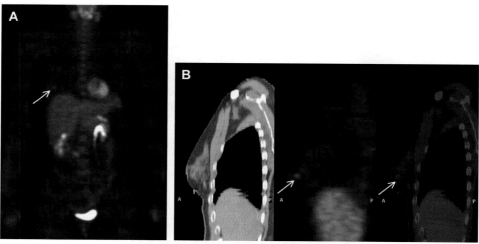

Fig. 3. Frontal maximum-intensity projection PET image (*A*) and sagittal slices from a PET/CT scan (*B*) show a mammographically occult 8-mm breast cancer detected incidentally by FDG-PET during a workup for presumed recurrent breast cancer in a patient with rising carcinoembryonic antigen. An ultrasound guided biopsy demonstrated an invasive ductal carcinoma, which was resected with clear margins.

A

B

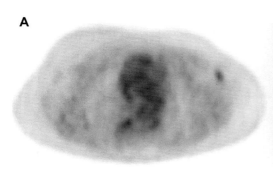
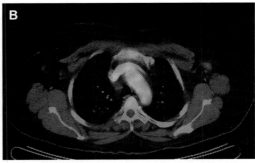

Fig. 4. Transaxial FDG-PET (*A*), and fused PET/CT image (*B*) with a small area of increased FDG uptake in a axillary lymph node metastasis.

Invasive lobular carcinomas were more often false-negative (65.2%) than invasive ductal carcinomas (23.7%). These results are consistent with a previous report from Crippa and colleagues [32], who found higher glucose metabolism for invasive ductal carcinomas (median SUV of 5.6) versus invasive lobular carcinomas (median SUV of 3.8). This is of particular importance in the clinical application of PET, because lobular carcinomas are more difficult to diagnose by imaging procedures such as mammography, sonography, and MRI [33–35]. The identification of multifocal or multicentric breast cancer plays an important role in the decision of therapy, because it limits breast-conserving surgery. Only 9 (50%) out of 18 patients who had multifocal or multicentric breast cancer were identified by PET [27]. Nevertheless, Schirrmeister and colleagues [29] found that PET was twice as sensitive in detecting multifocal lesions (sensitivity 63%, specificity 95%) than the combination of mammography and ultrasound (sensitivity 32%, specificity 93%).

The diagnosis of in-situ carcinomas has increased over the past decade, mainly due to increased use of and technological improvements in mammography. There is little information available about the ability of PET imaging to detect noninvasive breast cancer. Tse and coworkers [36] studied 14 patients and found that one out of two false-negative cases had predominantly intraductal cancer with microscopic invasive foci. In 12 patients, (10 DCIS and 2 LCIS) none out of six in-situ carcinomas smaller than 2 cm could be identified [27]. For larger in-situ carcinomas, three (50%) out of six displayed increased FDG uptake. Although the number of patients studied was small, these data suggest that PET imaging cannot contribute to an improved diagnosis of noninvasive breast cancer.

Vranjesevic and colleagues [37] evaluated the influence of the breast tissue density on FDG uptake of normal breast tissue, and found significantly lower SUVs for primarily fatty breasts than for dense breasts. Benign conditions of the breast are more common, and are often difficult to differentiate

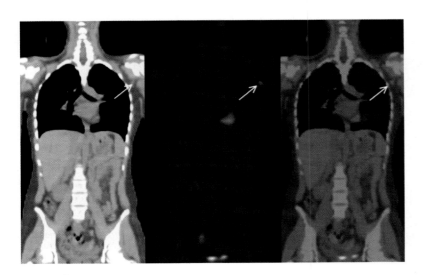

Fig. 5. Coronal PET/CT images demonstrate a false-positive axillary lymph node finding in a patient 2 weeks following a flu shot (*arrows*). There is also extensive, mild FDG uptake corresponding to metabolically active fat in the supraclavicular soft tissues.

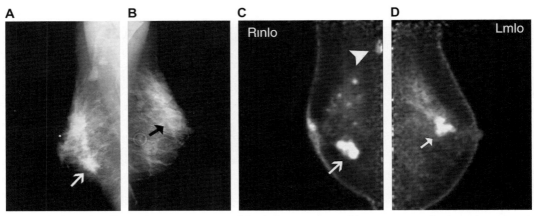

Fig. 6. Mediolateral radiograph mammograms of both breasts showed heterogeneously dense breast parenchyma with bilateral masses (*arrows*). Ultrasound-guided right breast biopsy showed invasive ductal carcinoma (*A, arrow*), whereas left breast ultrasound-guided biopsy showed papilloma (*B, arrow*). PEM of right breast showed dominant known invasive cancer (*C, arrow*) and smaller foci in upper breast, proving multicentric cancer with positive lymph node (*arrowhead*), and increased focal activity on left side (*D, arrow*) that was confirmed as DCIS at surgery.

from breast cancer in conventional imaging modalities. In general, benign breast masses display low FDG uptake. Only 3 out of 53 benign breast masses presented with focally increased tracer uptake, including one rare case of a ductal adenoma, one case with dysplastic tissue, and one fibroadenoma [27]. Fibroadenomas are common benign tumors, and only 1 out of 9 displayed increased tracer uptake. Moreover, dysplastic tissue often accounts for false-positive results in MRI, predominantly showing a diffuse pattern of little or moderate FDG uptake.

Biological features of breast cancer

FDG uptake in breast cancer shows considerable variation. To address that issue, the degree of tracer accumulation was recently correlated with various tumor characteristics [Table 2] [38]. Histologic sections of breast cancer specimens were analyzed for histologic type, microscopic tumor growth pattern, percentage of tumor cells, presence of inflammatory cells, density of blood vessels, histopathologic grading, tumor cell proliferation (mitotic rate and antibody binding of MIB-1), expression of estrogen and progesterone receptors, and expression of the glucose transporter protein Glut-1. Invasive ductal carcinomas displayed significantly higher FDG uptake compared with invasive lobular carcinomas. The SUVs for clearly defined lesions were higher compared with tumors with diffuse growth patterns. Lower densities of blood vessels corresponded to higher FDG uptakes. In addition, there was a positive correlation between FDG uptake and tumor cell proliferation, but only a weak relationship between FDG uptake and the percentage of tumor cells. There was no

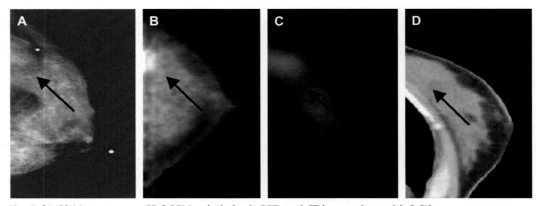

Fig. 7. (*A–D*) Mammogram, FDG-PEM, whole body PET, and CT in a patient with DCIS.

Table 1: **Sensitivity of FDG-PET and the size of breast cancer**

TNM	Size	n	Sensitivity
pTis		12	42%
pT1	<2.0 cm	44	68%
pT1a	<0.5 cm	4	25%
pT1b	>0.5–1.0 cm	8	25%
pT1c	>1.0–2.0 cm	32	84%
pT2	>2.0–5.0 cm	62	92%
	>2.0–3.0 cm	33	94%
	>3.0–4.0 cm	15	87%
	>4.0–5.0 cm	14	93%
pT3	>5.0 cm	14	100%

Data from Avril N, Rose CA, Schelling M, et al. Breast imaging with positron emission tomography and fluorine-18 fluorodeoxyglucose: use and limitations. J Clin Oncol 2000;18(20):3495–502.

relationship between FDG uptake and tumor size; axillary lymph node status; percentage of necrotic, fibrotic and cystic compounds; presence of inflammatory cells; steroid receptor status; and expression of Glut-1.

Histologic and immunohistochemical tissue analysis could not fully explain the variation of FDG uptake in breast cancer. The study authors concluded that the degree of metabolic changes in malignant tumors is mainly caused by complex interactions between the cellular energy metabolism and the microenvironment of the tumor. Hence FDG-PET uptake can not be used to predict the

Table 2: **FDG-uptake versus histology/immunohistochemistry**

SUV vs.	p	n
Histology (ductal versus lobular)	0.003	50
Tumor growth (nodular versus diffuse)	0.007	49
Grading	0.69	50
% tumor cells	0.06	50
Inflammatory cells	0.74	50
Capillaries	0.08	50
Proliferation (MIB-1)	0.009	40
Estrogen receptor status	0.47	42
Progesterone receptor status	0.29	42
Glut-1 transporter protein	0.21	45

Data from Avril N, Menzel M, Dose J, et al. Glucose metabolism of breast cancer assessed by 18F-FDG PET: histologic and immunohistochemical tissue analysis. J Nucl Med 2001;42(1):9–16.

biologic behaviors of breast cancer, such as differentiation, histopathologic grading, cell proliferation, or axillary lymph node status.

Loco-regional staging

The axillary lymph node status is still considered the single most important prognostic indicator in patients who have breast cancer. Clinical examination is generally unreliable for staging the axilla [39]. Lack of conventional imaging techniques to determine the axillary lymph node involvement with acceptable accuracy has been the main reason for axillary lymph node dissection; however, up to 70% of patients who have stage T1 and T2 tumors have negative axillary lymph nodes [40]. The extent, morbidity, and cost of the staging procedure of axillary lymph node dissection are often greater than those of the surgical treatment of the primary tumor. In anatomical based imaging modalities, such as computed tomography, ultrasound, and MRI, the size of a particular lymph node is of crucial importance to determine the tumor involvement. Generally, lymph node enlargement over 1 cm in diameter is the decisive criterion. In contrast, metabolic imaging with FDG-PET is suggested to provide more specific information, based on detecting increased glucose consumption of cancer tissue. In 1991, Wahl and coworkers [26] studied 12 patients who had locally advanced breast cancer, and found increased FDG uptake in axillary metastases. In 50 patients, Adler and colleagues [20] reported a sensitivity of 95%, a negative predictive value of 95%, and an overall accuracy of 77% for axillary PET imaging. Greco and coworkers [41] studied 167 consecutive breast cancer patients, and axillary involvement was detected in 68 of 72 patients, resulting in a sensitivity of 94.4% and a specificity of 86.3%; overall accuracy of lymph node staging with PET was 89.8%. There is some controversy about the sensitivity of axillary PET imaging, however [42]. It is a well-known phenomenon that the true FDG uptake is underestimated in small cancer deposits because of the limited spatial resolution of current PET devices, (approximately 6-8 mm). Therefore it cannot be expected that PET will provide visualization of micrometastases. Avril and colleagues [43] studied 51 patients and found overall sensitivity and specificity for detection of axillary lymph node metastases to be 79% and 96%, respectively. In patients who had primary breast tumors larger than 2 cm (>stage pT1), the sensitivity increased to 94%, with a corresponding specificity of 100%. PET could not identify lymph node metastases in 4 out of 6 patients who had small primary breast cancer (stage pT1), however, which led to a sensitivity of only 33% in this group.

Although the number of patients studied is small, this study clearly points out that the current achievable spatial resolution of PET imaging limits the detection of micrometastases and small tumor-infiltrated lymph nodes. This conclusion is also supported by others; for example, by Schirrmeister and coworkers [29], who studied 117 breast cancer patients and found similar results (sensitivity 79%, specificity 92%). In a prospective multicenter study representing the largest patient cohort so far [44], 360 women who had newly diagnosed invasive breast cancer underwent PET imaging. Three experienced readers blindly interpreted PET images, and the results from 308 axillae were compared with histopathology. If at least one probably or definitely abnormal axillary focus was considered positive, the sensitivity for PET was 61% and the specificity was 80%. Patients who had false-negative PET had significantly smaller and fewer tumor-positive lymph nodes than true-positive cases. Semiquantitative analysis of axillary FDG uptake showed that a nodal standardized uptake value (lean body mass) of more than 1.8 had a positive predictive value of 90% but a sensitivity of only 32%. Finding two or more intense foci of tracer uptake in the axilla was highly predictive of axillary metastasis, but had a sensitivity of only 27%.

Sentinel node biopsy has become accepted as a reliable method of predicting the status of the axilla in early stages of breast cancer [40]. There are few studies available directly comparing the diagnostic accuracy of PET with sentinel node biopsy in breast cancer patients. In one study [45], 5 out of 15 patients had sentinel lymph node metastases, but PET identified only 1 of these patients. The size of missed metastases ranged from a small micrometastasis identified only by immunohistochemistry to an 11-mm, tumor-involved lymph node. Another study [46] included 24 clinically node-negative breast cancer patients who had primary tumors smaller than 3 cm, and axillary staging by PET was accurate in 15 of 24 patients (62.5%). PET was false-negative in 8 of 10 node-positive patients, and false-positive in 1 patient. The sensitivity and specificity of FDG-PET were 20% and 93%, respectively. The mean diameter of false-negative axillary lymph node metastases was 7.5 mm, and ranged from 1 to 15 mm. In 32 breast cancer patients who had clinically negative axillary nodes, sentinel lymph node biopsy was false-negative in 1 patient, whereas PET missed lymph node metastases in 11 patients, resulting in a sensitivity of 20% [47]. These studies clearly indicate the limitation of FDG-PET for axillary staging of small primary tumors. FDG-PET is not accurate enough in clinically node-negative breast cancer patients qualifying for sentinel lymph node dissection. On the other hand, among patients who have larger tumors, sentinel biopsy can be avoided in those who have positive FDG-PET, in whom complete axillary lymph node dissection should be the primary procedure. FDG-PET cannot replace the axillary dissection, not only because of the limited sensitivity, but also because the number of involved lymph nodes and extranodal extension cannot be determined. In patients who have locally advanced disease and who are undergoing primary chemotherapy, however, FDG-PET seems to be a reliable method to determine the extent of disease.

Recently, the intrathoracic lymph node status has been retrospectively analyzed comparing CT and PET [48]. In 73 consecutive patients who had recurrent or metastatic disease, PET was able to correctly identify 40% of the patients who had intrathoracic lymph node metastases, resulting in a sensitivity of 85% and a specificity of 90%. Only 23% of the patients had suspiciously enlarged lymph nodes in CT, leading to a sensitivity of 54% and a specificity of 85%. PET and CT were both positive in 22% of the cases. Therefore overall diagnostic accuracy of PET was higher (88%) than that of CT (73%). Despite the limitation in detection of small tumor deposits, FDG-PET is currently the most sensitive imaging modality to detect lymph node metastases, including parasternal and mediastinal nodes.

Positron emission mammography

Because of the limited resolution of conventional PET scanners (4.8 to 7.1 mm in plane resolution), the even more limited resolution achieved with current clinical protocols (1 cm or greater), and the loss of contrast due to scatter, conventional PET scanners are unlikely to detect the small carcinomas that are detectable with other imaging modalities such as mammography and MRI. Dedicated breast PET—positron emission mammography (PEM)—was developed to improve both resolution and contrast of breast lesions and thereby improve small lesion detectability, while reducing the cost of imaging [49]. By optimizing scanner geometry for breast imaging, a dedicated breast PET scanner can achieve much higher resolution than a whole body scanner, while maintaining higher count sensitivity and a marked reduction in scatter [50,51]. Radiographic mammography uses compression to reduce the mean radiographic travel path, thereby reducing scatter. In an analogous manner, incorporating compression into PET imaging reduces the mean travel path of gamma emissions, with a resulting reduction in scatter. Because scatter represents such a low proportion of incident photons, septa or collimation is unnecessary, and a three-dimensional acquisition with full three-dimensional reconstruction is performed. An added benefit of compression is that images can be produced with a correspondence to radiograph mammograms, so PEM can be used to interrogate the functional status of abnormalities detected by mammography. Final output resolution of commercially available equipment is approximately 1.5 mm in plane. Resolution orthogonal to the imaging planes is dependant on the distance between the flat plate detectors (ie, the compressed thickness of the breast) and is generally not as good as in-plane resolution [52]. The dramatic improvement in resolution achieved results in the ability to detect smaller objects than would be detectable using a whole-body scanner (assuming identical object-to-background activity ratios) or to detect small objects with lower object-to-background activity ratios than would be detectable with whole body PET [19].

A recent multicenter study [52,53] demonstrated that high-resolution FDG-PEM detects in-situ components of cancers better than any other modality. This fact has been documented in retrospective surgical studies [52] as well as prospective imaging studies [53]. In the last-cited study, 93 consecutive subjects who had biopsy-proven breast cancer or suspicious breast lesions were recruited from four sites [53]. Only evaluable cases (eg, with proof of pathology) were shown to a blinded panel of imaging specialists for review. Patients who had Type I or poorly controlled Type II diabetes were excluded from participating in the study. Other diabetic patients were included, with the prospective decision that diagnostic performance of the PEM scans would be subsequently analyzed to determine whether diagnostic accuracy would differ in certain subsets of patients (eg, those who had diabetes or other medical conditions). Among index cancers in the 77 evaluable subjects reviewed, 39 (93%) out of 42 were PEM-positive. Including incidental lesions, 43 (90%) out of 48 malignancies were PEM-positive, including 10 (91%) out of 11 lesions of DCIS and 33 (89%) out of 37 invasive carcinomas. Three index malignancies (a 3-mm Grade II/III infiltrating and intraductal carcinoma, a 6-mm Grade I/III tubular carcinoma, and a 10-mm Grade I/III invasive ductal carcinoma with a positive axillary lymph node) were occult on FDG-PEM, but were visible mammographically. One contralateral 25-mm invasive lobular carcinoma was visible mammographically, but was only recognized by one of three PEM readers. Three DCIS foci (Grade II/III) were visible on FDG-PEM, but were mammographically occult. The combination of mammography, ultrasound, and FDG-PEM depicted 47 (98%) out of 48 cancers, with one case of contralateral Paget's disease caused by Grade II DCIS missed on all imaging modalities. FDG-PEM improved sensitivity when added to mammography, ultrasound, and clinical examination, without reducing accuracy.

One of three lesions with atypical ductal hyperplasia showed intense FDG uptake. Five (12%) of 41 other proven benign lesions showed intense FDG uptake, including two fibroadenomas, two fibrocystic changes, and one fat necrosis in a participant who had transverse rectus abdominis muscle (TRAM) flap reconstruction. The first two readers agreed on overall PEM assessment (ie, recommendation for biopsy or not) for 83% of the index lesions and 80% of the incidental lesions. Examining individual reader performance, at least one reader missed a malignancy in 8 index lesions and 3 incidental lesions. Examining all readings of index lesions, the average area under the receiver operating characteristic (ROC) curve was 0.91. Qualitatively high and asymmetric FDG uptake, as compared with radiograph mammograms, was the finding most predictive of malignancy. Although promising, additional prospective studies are needed to determine the clinical role of FDG-PEM imaging in the future.

Current clinical status of F-18 fluorodeoxyglucose-positron emission tomography in primary breast cancer

Breast cancer often displays only moderately increased FDG uptake, and considering the limited spatial resolution of FDG-PET, metabolic imaging results in a low sensitivity to detect small breast carcinomas, micrometastases, and small-tumor-infiltrated lymph nodes. The restricted sensitivity of FDG-PET does not allow the screening of asymptomatic women for breast cancer. Moreover, negative PET results in patients who have suspicious breast masses or abnormal mammography do not exclude breast cancer. Therefore, PET imaging may not be used as a routine application for evaluation of primary breast tumors, and currently cannot significantly reduce unnecessary invasive procedures in patients suspected of having breast cancer. Advances in technology such as the development of dedicated breast imaging devices (eg, PEM) may improve the detection of primary tumors with PET in the future. In patients who have locally advanced breast cancer, PET accurately determines the extent of disease, particularly the loco-regional lymph node status. In smaller tumors, the sentinel node biopsy has become the standard of care in many institutions.

References

[1] Sant M, Allemani C, Berrino F, et al. Breast carcinoma survival in Europe and the United States. Cancer 2004;100(4):715–22.

[2] Banerjee M, George J, Song EY, et al. Tree-based model for breast cancer prognostication. J Clin Oncol 2004;22(13):2567–75.

[3] Fitzgibbons PL, Page DL, Weaver D, et al. Prognostic factors in breast cancer. College of American Pathologists Consensus Statement 1999. Arch Pathol Lab Med 2000;124(7):966–78.

[4] Sickles EA. Breast masses: mammographic evaluation. Radiology 1989;173:297–303.

[5] Kopans DB, Feig SA. False positive rate of screening mammography. N Engl J Med 1998;339(8):562–4.

[6] Kopans DB. The positive predictive value of mammography. AJR Am J Roentgenol 1992;158:521–6.

[7] Liberman L, Menell JH. Breast imaging reporting and data system (BI-RADS). Radiol Clin North Am 2002;40(3):409–30, v.

[8] Meyer JE, Eberlein TJ, Stomper PC, et al. Biopsy of occult breast lesions. Analysis of 1261 abnormalities. JAMA 1990;263:2341–3.

[9] Sickles EA, Miglioretti DL, Ballard-Barbash R, et al. Performance benchmarks for diagnostic mammography. Radiology 2005;235(3):775–90.

[10] Bird RE, Wallace TW, Yankaskas BC. Analysis of cancer missed at screening mammography. Radiology 1992;184:613–7.

[11] Fine RE, Staren ED. Updates in breast ultrasound. Surg Clin North Am 2004;84(4):1001–34, v–vi.

[12] Mendelson EB. Problem-solving ultrasound. Radiol Clin North Am 2004;42(5):909–18, vii.

[13] Simmons R. Ultrasound in the changing approaches to breast cancer diagnosis and treatment. Breast J 2004;10(Suppl 1):S13–4.

[14] Lee CH. Problem solving MR imaging of the breast. Radiol Clin North Am 2004;42(5):919–34, vii.

[15] Hylton N. Magnetic resonance imaging of the breast: opportunities to improve breast cancer management. J Clin Oncol 2005;23(8):1678–84.

[16] Chen X, Moore MO, Lehman CD, et al. Combined use of MRI and PET to monitor response and assess residual disease for locally advanced breast cancer treated with neoadjuvant chemotherapy. Acad Radiol 2004;11(10):1115–24.

[17] Rohren EM, Turkington TG, Coleman RE. Clinical applications of PET in oncology. Radiology 2004;231(2):305–32.

[18] Brown RS, Wahl RL. Overexpression of Glut-1 glucose transporter in human breast cancer. An immunohistochemical study. Cancer 1993;72(10):2979–85.

[19] Adler LP, Crowe JP, al-Kaisi NK, et al. Evaluation of breast masses and axillary lymph nodes with [F-18] 2-deoxy-2-fluoro-D-glucose PET. Radiology 1993;187(3):743–50.

[20] Adler LP, Faulhaber PF, Schnur KC, et al. Axillary lymph node metastases: screening with [F-18]2-deoxy-2-fluoro-D-glucose (FDG) PET. Radiology 1997;203(2):323–7.

[21] Boerner AR, Weckesser M, Herzog H, et al. Optimal scan time for fluorine-18 fluorodeoxyglucose positron emission tomography in breast cancer. Eur J Nucl Med 1999;26(3):226–30.

[22] Avril N, Bense S, Ziegler SI, et al. Breast imaging with fluorine-18-FDG PET: quantitative image analysis. J Nucl Med 1997;38(8):1186–91.

[23] Stahl A, Weber WA, Avril N, et al. Effect of N-butylscopolamine on intestinal uptake of fluorine-18-fluorodeoxyglucose in PET imaging of the abdomen. Nuklearmedizin 2000;39(8):241–5.

[24] Minn H, Soini I. F-18 fluorodeoxyglucose scintigraphy in diagnosis and follow up of treatment in advanced breast cancer. Am J Clin Pathol 1989;91(5):535–41.

[25] Kubota K, Matsuzawa T, Amemiya A, et al. Imaging of breast cancer with F-18 fluorodeoxyglucose and positron emission tomography. J Comput Assist Tomogr 1989;13(6):1097–8.

[26] Wahl RL, Cody RL, Hutchins GD, et al. Primary and metastatic breast carcinoma: initial clinical evaluation with PET with the radiolabeled glucose analogue 2-[F-18]-fluoro-2-deoxy-D-glucose. Radiology 1991;179(3):765–70.

[27] Avril N, Rose CA, Schelling M, et al. Breast imaging with positron emission tomography and fluorine-18 fluorodeoxyglucose: use and limitations. J Clin Oncol 2000;18(20):3495–502.

[28] Avril N, Dose J, Jänicke F, et al. Metabolic characterization of breast tumors with positron emission tomography using F-18 fluorodeoxyglucose. J Clin Oncol 1996;14(6):1848–57.

[29] Schirrmeister H, Kuhn T, Guhlmann A, et al. Fluorine-18 2-deoxy-2-fluoro-D-glucose PET in the preoperative staging of breast cancer: comparison with the standard staging procedures. Eur J Nucl Med 2001;28(3):351–8.

[30] Goerres GW, Michel SC, Fehr MK, et al. Follow-up of women with breast cancer: comparison between MRI and FDG PET. Eur Radiol 2003;13(7):1635–44.

[31] Baslaim MM, Bakheet SM, Bakheet R, et al. 18-Fluorodeoxyglucose-positron emission tomography in inflammatory breast cancer. World J Surg 2003;27(10):1099–104.

[32] Crippa F, Seregni E, Agresti R, et al. Association between F-18 fluorodeoxyglucose uptake and postoperative histopathology, hormone receptor status, thymidine labelling index and p53 in primary breast cancer: a preliminary observation. Eur J Nucl Med 1998;25(10):1429–34.

[33] Krecke KN, Gisvold JJ. Invasive lobular carcinoma of the breast: mammographic findings and extent of disease at diagnosis in 184 patients. AJR Am J Roentgenol 1993;161(5):957–60.

[34] Gilles R, Guinebretière J-M, Lucidarme O, et al. Nonpalpable breast tumors: diagnosis with contrast-enhanced subtraction dynamic MR imaging. Radiology 1994;191:625–31.

[35] Paramagul CP, Helvie MA, Adler DD. Invasive lobular carcinoma: sonographic appearance

and role of sonography in improving diagnostic sensitivity. Radiology 1995;195(1):231–4.

[36] Tse NY, Hoh CK, Hawkins RA, et al. The application of positron emission tomographic imaging with fluorodeoxyglucose to the evaluation of breast disease. Ann Surg 1992;216(1):27–34.

[37] Vranjesevic D, Schiepers C, Silverman DH, et al. Relationship between 18F-FDG uptake and breast density in women with normal breast tissue. J Nucl Med 2003;44(8):1238–42.

[38] Avril N, Menzel M, Dose J, et al. Glucose metabolism of breast cancer assessed by 18F-FDG PET: histologic and immunohistochemical tissue analysis. J Nucl Med 2001;42(1):9–16.

[39] Sacre RA. Clinical evaluation of axillar lymph nodes compared to surgical and pathological findings. Eur J Surg Oncol 1986;12(2):169–73.

[40] Veronesi U, Paganelli G, Galimberti V, et al. Sentinel-node biopsy to avoid axillary dissection in breast cancer with clinically negative lymph-nodes. Lancet 1997;349(9069):1864–7.

[41] Greco M, Crippa F, Agresti R, et al. Axillary lymph node staging in breast cancer by 2-Fluoro-2-deoxy-D-glucose-positron emission tomography: Clinical evaluation and alternative management. J Natl Cancer Inst 2001;93(8):630–5.

[42] Torrenga H, Licht J, van der Hoeven JJ, et al. Re: axillary lymph node staging in breast cancer by 2-fluoro-2-deoxy-D-glucose-positron emission tomography: clinical evaluation and alternative management. J Natl Cancer Inst 2001;93(21):1659–61.

[43] Avril N, Dose J, Jänicke F, et al. Assessment of axillary lymph node involvement in breast cancer patients with positron emission tomography using radiolabeled 2-(fluorine-18)-fluoro-2-deoxy-D-glucose. J Natl Cancer Inst 1996;88(17):1204–9.

[44] Wahl RL, Siegel BA, Coleman RE, et al. Prospective multicenter study of axillary nodal staging by positron emission tomography in breast cancer: a report of the staging breast cancer with PET Study Group. J Clin Oncol 2004;22(2):277–85.

[45] Kelemen PR, Lowe V, Phillips N. Positron emission tomography and sentinel lymph node dissection in breast cancer. Clin Breast Cancer 2002;3(1):73–7.

[46] Fehr MK, Hornung R, Varga Z, et al. Axillary staging using positron emission tomography in breast cancer patients qualifying for sentinel lymph node biopsy. Breast J 2004;10(2):89–93.

[47] Barranger E, Grahek D, Antoine M, et al. Evaluation of fluorodeoxyglucose positron emission tomography in the detection of axillary lymph node metastases in patients with early-stage breast cancer. Ann Surg Oncol 2003;10(6):622–7.

[48] Eubank WB, Mankoff DA, Takasugi J, et al. 18fluorodeoxyglucose positron emission tomography to detect mediastinal or internal mammary metastases in breast cancer. J Clin Oncol 2001;19(15):3516–23.

[49] Murthy K, Aznar M, Thompson CJ, et al. Results of preliminary clinical trials of the positron emission mammography system PEM-I: a dedicated breast imaging system producing glucose metabolic images using FDG. J Nucl Med 2000;41(11):1851–8.

[50] Bergman AM, Thompson CJ, Murthy K, et al. Technique to obtain positron emission mammography images in registration with x-ray mammograms. Med Phys 1998;25(11):2119–29.

[51] Weinberg I, Majewski S, Weisenberger A, et al. Preliminary results for positron emission mammography: real-time functional breast imaging in a conventional mammography gantry. Eur J Nucl Med 1996;23(7):804–6.

[52] Weinberg IN, Beylin D, Zavarzin V, et al. Positron emission mammography: high-resolution biochemical breast imaging. Technol Cancer Res Treat 2005;4(1):55–60.

[53] Tafra L, Cheng Z, Uddo O, et al. Pilot clinical trial of FDG positron emission mammography (PEM) in the surgical management of breast cancer. Am J Surg 2005;190:628–32.

RADIOLOGIC
CLINICS
OF NORTH AMERICA

Radiol Clin N Am 45 (2007) 659–667

ELSEVIER
SAUNDERS

Diagnosis of Recurrent and Metastatic Disease Using F-18 Fluorodeoxyglucose-Positron Emission Tomography in Breast Cancer

William B. Eubank, MD

Breast cancer is the most common non-skin cancer, and the second leading cause of cancer death in women [1]. There are 40,000 women per year dying of breast cancer in the United States, and most breast cancer victims die of progressive metastatic disease [1]. Because optimal treatment of patients who have recurrent breast cancer depends on knowing the true extent of disease, accurate staging of these patients is an important public health problem. This is a useful application of FDG-PET when it is performed to complement conventional imaging (CI) such as CT, MRI, and bone scintigraphy. The additional metabolic information provided by FDG-PET increases the accuracy of detecting recurrent or metastatic lesions [2–12]. This is particularly true in the evaluation of anatomic

regions that have been previously treated by surgery or radiation [13], in which the discrimination between post-treatment scar and recurrent tumor can be problematic. FDG-PET can also significantly impact the choice of treatment, especially in patients who have more advanced or recurrent disease [14,15].

The recognition that breast cancer is a systemic disease, even in its early stages, led to the current approach to treatment, which combines local measures such as surgery and radiotherapy with systemic treatment [16]. For most clinical trial studies, local failure is defined as any recurrence of tumor in the ipsilateral chest wall or mastectomy scar; regional failure is defined as any recurrence of tumor in the ipsilateral supraclavicular, infraclavicular,

This article was previously published in PET Clinics 2006;1:15–24.
This work was supported in part by National Institutes of Health (NIH) grants RO1CA42045, RO1CA72064, RO1CA90771, and S10RR177229.
Department of Radiology, Puget Sound Veterans Administration Health Care System, 1660 South Columbian Way, Seattle, WA 98108-1597, USA
E-mail address: weubank@u.washington.edu

doi:10.1016/j.rcl.2007.05.005

axillary, or internal mammary nodes; and recurrence of tumor in any other site is considered as distant failure [17]. In general, systemic therapy is used at almost all disease stages; however, isolated loco-regional disease or single sites of metastatic recurrence are also treated with surgery and radiation therapy [18,19]. It is hoped that the potential of FDG-PET to provide more accurate and earlier detection of breast cancer recurrences will translate into more effective treatment strategies and better health outcomes for these patients in the future.

Loco-regional recurrence

Recurrence in the breast, skin of the breast, axillary nodes, chest wall, and supraclavicular nodes are the most common sites of first loco-regional recurrence after primary surgical resection [20,21]. The shift toward breast-conserving surgery and local radiation therapy for early breast cancer in recent years has heightened concern over loco-regional recurrence [22]. The incidence of loco-regional recurrence after breast conservation treatment ranges from 5% to 22% [23]. Independent risk factors associated with loco-regional recurrence in this group of patients include positive margins at surgical resection, tumors with extensive intraductal component, high grade ductal carcinoma in situ (DCIS), patient age under 40 years, and absence

of radiation after breast conservation therapy [23,24].

Among patients treated with mastectomy, axillary node dissection, and adjuvant chemotherapy, the most common sites of loco-regional recurrence are the chest wall (68% of loco-regional recurrences) and supraclavicular nodes (41% of loco-regional recurrences) [Fig. 1] [25]. Recurrent disease at both of these sites is associated with poor prognosis in terms of survival after recurrence [26–28]. Factors that predict an increased risk of chest wall or supraclavicular node recurrence include four or more positive axillary nodes, tumor size 4 cm or larger, and extranodal extension of 2 mm or more [25]. Supraclavicular node recurrence is technically considered Stage IV disease, and is generally considered a harbinger to more widely disseminated disease; however, patients who have supraclavicular node involvement as the sole site of disseminated disease may benefit from aggressive local radiotherapy.

One clinical situation where FDG-PET has been shown to be helpful is in the evaluation of previously treated patients who have symptoms of brachial plexopathy. This debilitating condition can be secondary to tumor recurrence in the axilla or chest wall, or caused by scarring of tissue neighboring the brachial plexus from previous surgery or radiation. Because the signs and symptoms of loco-regional recurrence often overlap with the side

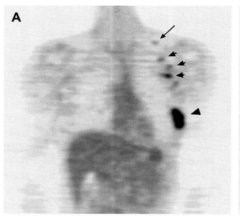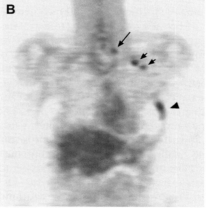

Fig. 1. A 49-year-old woman who underwent bilateral mastectomies and reconstruction with implants 7 years before recurrence of disease. She originally had extensive lobular carcinoma in situ with two small (2–3 mm) foci of invasive lobular carcinoma in the right breast. Sentinel node and limited low axillary lymph node dissection revealed no pathologically involved nodes, and surgical margins were negative. She received no adjuvant treatment, but opted for prophylactic left mastectomy. At time of recurrence, she presented with palpable left chest wall mass (biopsy-proven invasive ductal carcinoma) and axillary nodes. Coronal FDG-PET image (*A*) shows recurrent chest wall mass (*arrowhead*; standardized uptake value [SUV] = 8.2) lateral to breast implant, uptake in several axillary nodes (*small arrows*; maximum SUV = 4.5), and left supraclavicular node (*long arrow*; SUV = 2.1). At more anterior level, coronal FDG-PET image (*B*) shows uptake in a left internal mammary node (*long arrow*; SUV = 2.0) in addition to uptake in left axillary nodes (*short arrows*) and the left breast (*arrowhead*).

effects of treatment [29,30] and patients who have tumor recurrence may benefit from surgical resection [31,32], it is important to distinguish one from the other. Hathaway and colleagues [33] showed the value of combining the functional information of FDG-PET and the anatomic information from dedicated MRI to decide whether patients would benefit from further surgery. Other studies [34] have confirmed these early findings.

Intrathoracic lymphatic recurrences

Lymphatic drainage to the internal mammary nodal chain is an important pathway of spread of disease, both at the time of initial diagnosis and after primary treatment of breast cancer. Data from sentinel node lymphoscintigraphy series in patients who had early breast cancer at the author's institution reveal that overall prevalence of drainage to the internal mammary nodes is 17% [35]. This is a similar prevalence to that shown in early extended radical mastectomy series [36–38], in which metastasis to internal mammary nodes occurred in close to one in five women who had operable (Stage II–III) breast cancer. Metastasis to internal mammary nodes can occur from tumor located anywhere in the breast; however, in the series of the author and colleagues, internal mammary drainage was significantly less frequent in tumors located in the upper outer quadrant (10%) compared with the other three quadrants and subareolar portion of the breast (17%–29%) [35]. Metastasis to the internal mammary and axillary nodes usually occurs synchronously but infrequently (4%–6% incidence) may be isolated to the internal mammary chain [36,39]. The prognosis of patients who have internal mammary and axillary nodal metastasis is significantly worse compared with patients who have only axillary node disease [40,41], suggesting that internal mammary nodal chain is a conduit for more widespread dissemination of disease.

The importance of internal mammary nodal detection and treatment remains controversial [42]. Unlike axillary nodes, internal mammary nodes are not routinely biopsied as part of an individual patient's staging work-up, and their status is generally unknown. There has been reluctance to biopsy internal mammary nodes because: (1) early radiotherapy trials (before the era of routine adjuvant chemotherapy) failed to demonstrate a clear benefit in survival with internal mammary chain radiation, and (2) there is a relatively high complication risk (pneumothorax and bleeding) associated with internal mammary nodal sampling. A recent large, prospective, randomized, radiotherapy trial [43] has shown a benefit in systemic relapse-free and overall survival from aggressive regional nodal irradiation (including internal mammary field) following lumpectomy or mastectomy, even in patients who had fairly limited spread to the axilla. These data suggest that eradication of residual loco-regional metastasis (including internal mammary nodal disease) has a strong systemic effect.

FDG uptake in the internal mammary nodal chain has been anecdotally reported in some of the studies that have focused on detection of primary tumor or axillary staging [44,45]. In one study of 85 patients who underwent FDG-PET before axillary node dissection [44], 12 (14%) had uptake in the internal mammary region, but there was no histological confirmation of these nodes. The author and colleagues' experience with imaging patients who have locally advanced breast cancer shows that the prevalence of internal mammary FDG uptake can be as high as 25%, and that the presence of internal mammary FDG uptake predicts treatment failure patterns of disease consistent with internal mammary nodal involvement and progression [Fig. 2] [46]. A preliminary study by Bernstein and coworkers [47] showed the feasibility of detecting internal mammary nodal metastases in early-stage patients using FDG-PET. FDG-PET may prove to be an ideal method of noninvasively staging this important nodal region, and may aid in the selection of patients who would potentially benefit most from directed internal mammary nodal radiotherapy; however, further work needs to be done to confirm FDG-PET findings with histopathology.

Neoplastic spread to mediastinal nodes is also common in patients who have advanced disease, and the mediastinum is a common site of recurrence in patients who have undergone axillary node dissection and radiation [Fig. 3]. As with internal mammary nodes, mediastinal nodes are rarely sampled in breast cancer patients. CT, the conventional method of staging these nodes, relies on size criteria to determine the presence or absence of disease. This method has been proven significantly less accurate than FDG-PET in patients who have non-small–cell lung cancer in which histologic analysis is used as the gold standard [48,49]. In the author and colleagues' retrospective series of 73 patients who had recurrent or metastatic breast cancer and who underwent both FDG-PET and chest CT [50], FDG uptake in mediastinal or internal mammary nodes was two times more prevalent than suspiciously enlarged nodes by CT, suggesting that PET is a much more sensitive technique at detecting nodal disease. In the subset of patients who had confirmation, the sensitivity of

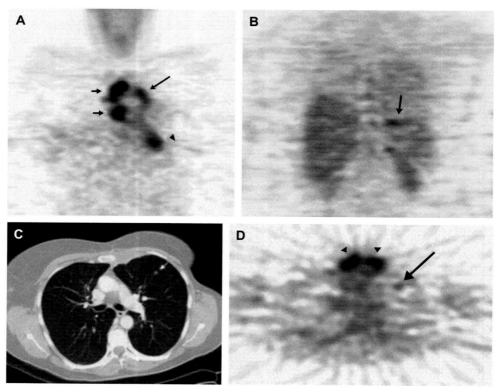

Fig. 2. A 46-year-old woman who presented with sternal pain 5 years after undergoing left mastectomy for invasive ductal carcinoma (T3, N0) followed by chemotherapy and radiation. Anterior coronal FDG-PET image (*A*) shows intense uptake in the left parasternal region (*long arrow*) and sternum (*short arrows*; maximum SUV = 9.4) consistent with disease in the internal mammary node chain with local spread to the sternum. Physiologic uptake in the anterior heart (*arrowhead*) is also present. A posterior coronal FDG-PET image of the chest (*B*) shows linear uptake along the supradiaphragmatic region (*arrow*; SUV = 4.1) consistent with pleural metastasis and axial FDG-PET (*C*) and CT (*D*) of the upper chest show a small lung metastasis (*arrows*; SUV = 2.0) in addition to sternal uptake (*arrowheads*).

FDG-PET was significantly higher (85%) than CT (50%), with nearly the same level of specificity (90% for PET and 83% for CT). Ten of 33 (30%) patients suspected of having only loco-regional recurrence by CI and clinical examination had mediastinal or internal mammary FDG uptake. Risk factors associated with mediastinal or internal mammary FDG uptake in these patients were recurrent chest wall invasion and three or more positive axillary nodes.

Distant metastases

The skeleton is the most common site of distant metastasis in breast cancer; nearly 70% of patients who have advanced disease have bone metastasis [51]. Bone scintigraphy is considered the most sensitive method of detecting and determining the extent of skeletal metastases; however, purely osteolytic lesions or metastases confined to the marrow

cavity may be difficult to detect on bone scintigraphy, because of a lack of sufficient osteoblastic response [52]. Retrospective studies comparing the sensitivity of bone scintigraphy to FDG-PET in the detection of skeletal metastases in patients who have advanced disease have shown conflicting results [3,4,9,53–56]. Some studies have shown FDG-PET to be equal or superior to planar bone scintigraphy in the detection of skeletal metastases [53,54], whereas others have shown FDG-PET to be less sensitive [3,4,9,55] on a lesion-based analysis. The results from a study by Cook and colleagues [56], in which skeletal metastases from breast cancer patients were categorized into osteoblastic, osteolytic, or mixed disease subsets based on plain film or CT findings, provides an explanation for these conflicting reports. In the study of 23 breast cancer patients who had known skeletal metastases and who underwent both bone scintigraphy and FDG-PET, FDG-PET detected more

breast cancer benefit the most from FDG-PET. A previous investigation [14] showed that FDG-PET had a major impact on the management of patients who had breast cancer and who underwent restaging for local or distant recurrences. FDG-PET changed the clinical stage in 36% of patients and induced changes in therapy in 58% of the patients. In the author and colleagues' retrospective study of 125 patients who had advanced breast cancer and who were undergoing CI and FDG-PET for staging [15], the extent of disease was changed in 67% of patients (increased in 43% and decreased in 24%), and the therapeutic plan was altered in 32% of patients based on FDG-PET findings. FDG-PET altered therapy most frequently in two subgroups of patients: (1) patients who had suspected or proven loco-regional recurrence, under consideration for aggressive local therapy (FDG-PET altered treatment in 44%), and (2) patients who had known metastases being evaluated for response to therapy (FDG-PET altered treatment in 33%). These results indicate that FDG-PET should not be used as the sole restaging tool in patients who have recurrent or metastatic disease, but should be used to answer specific questions that will likely impact their management. Future prospective trials using oncologist-directed questionnaires will help to further define the role and provide data for the cost-benefit analysis of FDG-PET in staging patients who have advanced breast cancer.

There have been a few preliminary studies showing promise for FDG-PET/CT in the evaluation of patients who have recurrent or metastatic breast cancer [61–63]. Because of the accurate registration of metabolic and morphologic images from these integrated systems, the accuracy in localizing FDG uptake is improved; this can potentially lead to an improvement in specificity (reduction in false positive results) and staging of disease compared with separate evaluation of CT and PET data. PET/CT also shows promise in radiation treatment planning by modifying target tissue volumes selected for irradiation, based on the combination of morphologic and metabolic data [64]. The impact of PET/CT on patient outcomes needs to be addressed in future studies.

Summary

FDG-PET is a useful tool in the evaluation of patients who have suspected or proven breast cancer recurrence. In the clinical setting, it should be used as a complement to conventional staging studies and not as a replacement. FDG-PET is generally more sensitive in the detection of loco-regional and distant metastases than conventional imaging, and is therefore a more accurate method of determining the true extent of disease. One exception is the detection of sclerotic bone metastases; these lesions are often not metabolically active enough for FDG-PET detection, but are readily detected by bone scintigraphy. To have the greatest impact on patient management, FDG-PET should be used to answer specific clinical questions. In the clinical setting of an asymptomatic patient who has rising tumor markers and negative or equivocal findings on clinical examination or CI, FDG-PET has the ability to detect otherwise occult disease. Preliminary investigations show that FDG-PET has the greatest impact on the choice of treatment in patients who have suspected or proven loco-regional recurrence and who are being considered for aggressive curative treatment, and in the evaluation of treatment response in patients who have metastatic disease.

Acknowledgments

The authors wish to acknowledge Erin Schubert for help with figure reproduction.

References

[1] Greenlee RT, Murray T, Bolden S, et al. Cancer Statistics, 2000. CA Cancer J Clin 2000;50(1):7–33.

[2] Bender H, Kirst J, Palmedo H, et al. Value of ^{18}fluoro-deoxyglucose positron emission tomography in the staging of recurrent breast carcinoma. Anticancer Res 1997;17(3B):1687–92.

[3] Moon DH, Maddahi J, Silverman DHS, et al. Accuracy of whole-body [fluorine-18]-FDG-PET for the detection of recurrent or metastatic breast carcinoma. J Nucl Med 1998;39(3):431–5.

[4] Lonneux M, Borbath I, Berliere M, et al. The place of whole-body FDG-PET for the diagnosis of distant recurrence of breast cancer. Clin Positron Imaging 2000;3(2):45–9.

[5] Kim TS, Moon WK, Lee DS, et al. Fluorodeoxyglucose positron emission tomography for detection of recurrent or metastatic breast cancer. World J Surg 2001;25(7):829–34.

[6] Lin WY, Tsai SC, Cheng KY, et al. Fluorine-18 FDG-PET in detecting local recurrence and distant metastasis in breast cancer–Taiwanese experiences. Cancer Invest 2002;20(5–6):725–9.

[7] Liu CS, Shen YY, Lin CC, et al. Clinical impact of [18F]FDG-PET in patients with suspected recurrent breast cancer based on asymptomatically elevated tumor marker serum levels: a preliminary report. Jpn J Clin Oncol 2002;32(7):244–7.

[8] Suarez M, Perez-Castejon MJ, Jimenez A, et al. Early diagnosis of recurrent breast cancer with FDG-PET in patients with progressive elevation of serum tumor markers. Q J Nucl Med 2002; 46(2):113–21.

[9] Gallowitsch HJ, Kresnik E, Gasser J, et al. [18F]-fluorodeoxyglucose positron-emission tomography in the diagnosis of tumor recurrence and

metastases in the follow-up of patients with breast carcinoma: a comparison to conventional imaging. Invest Radiol 2003;38(5):250–6.

[10] Siggelkow W, Zimny M, Faridi A, et al. The value of positron emission tomography in the follow-up for breast cancer. Anticancer Res 2003; 23(2C):1859–68.

[11] Kamel EM, Wyss MT, Fehr MK, et al. [18F]-fluoro-deoxyglucose positron emission tomography in patients with suspected recurrence of breast cancer. J Cancer Res Clin Oncol 2003;129(3):147–53.

[12] Eubank WB, Mankoff DA, Vesselle HJ, et al. Detection of locoregional and distant recurrences in breast cancer patients by using FDG-PET. Radiographics 2002;22(1):5–17.

[13] Eubank WB, Mankoff DA, Schmiedl UP, et al. Imaging of oncologic patients: benefit of combined CT and [F-18]-fluorodeoxyglucose positron emission tomography scan interpretation in the diagnosis of malignancy. Am J Roentgenol 1998;171(4):1103–10.

[14] Yap CS, Seltzer MA, Schiepers C, et al. Impact of whole-body ^{18}FDG-PET on staging and managing patients with breast cancer: the referring physician's perspective. J Nucl Med 2001;42(9): 1334–7.

[15] Eubank WB, Mankoff DA, Bhattacharya M, et al. Impact of [F-18]-Fluorodeoxyglucose PET on defining the extent of disease and management of patients with recurrent or metastatic breast cancer. Am J Roentgenol 2004;83(2):479–86.

[16] Hortobagyi GN. Developments in chemotherapy of breast cancer. Cancer 2000;88(Suppl 12): 3073–9.

[17] Taghian A, Jeong J, Mamounas E, et al. Patterns of locoregional failure in patients with operable breast cancer treated by mastectomy and adjuvant chemotherapy with or without tamoxifen and without radiotherapy: results from five National Surgical Adjuvant Breast and Bowel Project randomized clinical trials. J Clin Oncol 2004;22(21):4247–54.

[18] Schwaibold F, Fowble BL, Solin LJ, et al. The results of radiation therapy for isolated local regional recurrence after mastectomy. Int J Radiat Oncol Biol Phys 1991;21(2):299–310.

[19] Probstfeld MR, O'Connell TX. Treatment of locally recurrent breast carcinoma. Arch Surg 1989;124(10):1127–9 [discussion: 1130].

[20] Valagussa P, Bonadonna G, Veronesi U. Patterns of relapse and survival following radical mastectomy. Analysis of 716 consecutive patients. Cancer 1978;41(3):1170–8.

[21] Kamby C, Rose C, Ejlertsen B, et al. Stage and pattern of metastases in patients with breast cancer. Eur J Cancer Clin Oncol 1987;23(12): 1925–34.

[22] Schmolling J, Maus B, Rezek D, et al. Breast preservation versus mastectomy—recurrence and survival rates of primary breast cancer patients treated at the UFK Bonn. Eur J Gynaecol Oncol 1997;18(1):29–33.

[23] Huston TL, Simmons RM. Locally recurrent breast cancer after conservation therapy. Am J Surg 2005;189(2):229–35.

[24] Leborgne F, Leborgne JH, Ortega B, et al. Breast conservation treatment of early stage breast cancer: patterns of failure. Int J Radiat Oncol Biol Phys 1995;31(4):765–75.

[25] Katz A, Strom EA, Buchholz TA, et al. Locoregional recurrence patterns after mastectomy and doxorubicin-based chemotherapy: implications for postoperative irradiation. J Clin Oncol 2000;18(15):2817–27.

[26] Aristei C, Marsella AR, Chionne F, et al. Regional node failure in patients with four or more positive lymph nodes submitted to conservative surgery followed by radiotherapy to the breast. Am J Clin Oncol 2000;23(3):217–21.

[27] Nikkanen TA. Recurrence of breast cancer. A retrospective study of 569 cases in clinical Stages I–III. Acta Chir Scand 1981;147(4):239–45.

[28] Kiricuta IC, Willner J, Kolbl O, et al. The prognostic significance of the supraclavicular lymph node metastases in breast cancer patients. Int J Radiat Oncol Biol Phys 1994;28(2):387–93.

[29] Iyer RB, Fenstermacher MJ, Libshitz HI. MR imaging of the treated brachial plexus. Am J Roentgenol 1996;167(1):225–9.

[30] Bagley FH, Walsh JW, Cady B, et al. Carcinomatous versus radiation-induced brachial plexus neuropathy in breast cancer. Cancer 1978;41(6): 2154–7.

[31] Toi M, Tanaka S, Bando M, et al. Outcome of surgical resection for chest wall recurrence in breast cancer patients. J Surg Oncol 1997;37(1): 853–63.

[32] Hathaway CL, Rand RP, Moe R, et al. Salvage surgery for locally advanced and locally recurrent breast cancer. Arch Surg 1994;129(6):582–7.

[33] Hathaway PB, Mankoff DA, Maravilla KR, et al. The value of combined FDG-PET and magnetic resonance imaging in the evaluation of suspected recurrent local-regional breast cancer: preliminary experience. Radiology 1998;210(3): 807–14.

[34] Ahmad A, Barrington S, Maisey M, et al. Use of positron emission tomography in evaluation of brachial plexopathy in breast cancer patients. Br J Cancer 1999;79(3–4):478–82.

[35] Byrd DR, Dunnwald LK, Mankoff DA, et al. Internal mammary lymph node drainage patterns with breast cancer documented by breast lymphoscintigraphy. J Surg Oncol 2001;8(3): 234–40.

[36] Donegan WL. The influence of untreated internal mammary metastases upon the course of mammary cancer. Cancer 1977;39(2):533–8.

[37] Veronesi U, Cascinelli N, Greco M, et al. Prognosis of breast cancer patients after mastectomy and dissection of internal mammary nodes. Ann Surg 1985;202(6):702–7.

[38] Lacour J, Le M, Caceres E, et al. Radical mastectomy versus radical mastectomy plus internal

mammary dissection. Ten year results of an international cooperative trial in breast cancer. Cancer 1983;51(10):1941–3.

[39] Noguchi M, Ohta N, Thomas M, et al. Risk of internal mammary lymph node metastases and its prognostic value in breast cancer patients. J Surg Oncol 1993;52(1):26–30.

[40] Veronesi U, Marubini E, Del Vecchio M, et al. Local recurrences and distant metastases after conservative breast cancer treatments: partly independent events. J Natl Cancer Inst 1995; 87(1):19–27.

[41] Cody HS 3rd, Urban JA. Internal mammary node status: a major prognosticator in axillary node-negative breast cancer. Ann Surg Oncol 1995; 2(1):32–7.

[42] Freedman GM, Fowble BL, Nicolaou N, et al. Should internal mammary lymph nodes in breast cancer be a target for the radiation oncologist? Int J Radiat Oncol Biol Phys 2000;46(4):805–14.

[43] Ragaz J, Olivotto IA, Spinelli JJ, et al. Locoregional radiation therapy in patients with high-risk breast cancer receiving adjuvant chemotherapy: 20-year results of the British Columbia randomized trial. J Natl Cancer Inst 2005;97(2):116–25.

[44] Schirrmeister H, Kuhn T, Guhlmann A, et al. [F-18]-2-deoxy-2-fluoro-D-glucose PET in the preoperative staging of breast cancer: comparison with the standard staging procedures. Eur J Nucl Med 2001;28(3):351–8.

[45] Greco M, Crippa F, Agresti R, et al. Axillary lymph node staging in breast cancer by 2-fluoro-2-deoxy-D-glucose-positron emission tomography: clinical evaluation and alternative management. J Natl Cancer Inst 2001;93(8):630–5.

[46] Bellon JR, Livingston RB, Eubank WB, et al. Evaluation of the internal mammary (IM) lymph nodes by FDG-PET in locally advanced breast cancer (LABC). Am J Clin Oncol 2004;27(4):407–10.

[47] Bernstein V, Jones A, Mankoff DA, et al. Assessment of internal mammary lymph nodes by fluorodeoxyglucose positron emission (FDG-PET) in medial hemisphere breast cancer. [abstract]. J Nucl Med 2000;41:289P.

[48] Vansteenkiste JF, Stroobants SG, De Leyn PR, et al. Lymph node staging in non-small–cell lung cancer with FDG-PET scan: a prospective study on 690 lymph node stations from 68 patients. J Clin Oncol 1998;16(6):2142–9.

[49] Scott WJ, Gobar LS, Terry JD, et al. Mediastinal lymph node staging of non-small–cell lung cancer: a prospective comparison of computed tomography and positron emission tomography. J Thorac Cardiovasc Surg 1996;111(3):642–8.

[50] Eubank WB, Mankoff DA, Takasugi J, et al. [18]Fluorodeoxyglucose positron emission tomography to detect mediastinal or internal mammary metastases in breast cancer. J Clin Oncol 2001; 19(15):3516–23.

[51] Coleman RE, Rubens RD. The clinical course of bone metastases from breast cancer. Br J Cancer 1987;55(1):61–6.

[52] Nielsen OS, Munro AJ, Tannock IF. Bone metastases: pathophysiology and management policy. J Clin Oncol 1991;9(3):509–24.

[53] Ohta M, Tokuda Y, Suzuki Y, et al. Whole body PET for the evaluation of bony metastases in patients with breast cancer: comparison with 99Tcm-MDP bone scintigraphy. Nucl Med Commun 2001;22(8):875–9.

[54] Yang SN, Liang JA, Lin FJ, et al. Comparing whole body [18F]-2-deoxyglucose positron emission tomography and technetium-99m methylene diphosphonate bone scan to detect bone metastases in patients with breast cancer. J Cancer Res Clin Oncol 2002;128(6):325–8.

[55] Kao CH, Hsieh JF, Tsai SC, et al. Comparison and discrepancy of [18F]-2-deoxyglucose positron emission tomography and Tc-99m MDP bone scan to detect bone metastases. Anticancer Res 2000;20(3B):2189–92.

[56] Cook GJ, Houston S, Rubens R, et al. Detection of bone metastases in breast cancer by [18]FDG-PET: differing metabolic activity in osteoblastic and osteolytic lesions. J Clin Oncol 1998;16(10): 3375–9.

[57] Uematsu T, Yuen S, Yukisawa S, et al. Comparison of FDG-PET and SPECT for detection of bone metastases in breast cancer. Am J Roentgenol 2005;84(4):1266–73.

[58] Schirrmeister H, Guhlmann A, Kotzerke J, et al. Early detection and accurate description of extent of metastatic bone disease in breast cancer with fluoride ion and positron emission tomography. J Clin Oncol 1999;17(8): 2381–9.

[59] Schirrmeister H, Glatting G, Hetzel J, et al. Prospective evaluation of the clinical value of planar bone scans, SPECT, and ^{18}F-labeled NaF PET in newly diagnosed lung cancer. J Nucl Med 2001;42(12):1800–4.

[60] Vranjesevic D, Filmont JE, Meta J, et al. Whole-body ^{18}F-FDG-PET and conventional imaging for predicting outcome in previously treated breast cancer patients. J Nucl Med 2002;43(3): 325–9.

[61] Pelosi E, Messa C, Sironi S, et al. Value of integrated PET/CT for lesion localisation in cancer patients: a comparative study. Eur J Nucl Med Mol Imaging 2004;31(7):932–9.

[62] Buck AK, Wahl A, Eicher U, et al. Combined morphological and functional imaging with FDG-PET/CT for restaging breast cancer—impact on patient management. [abstract]. J Nucl Med 2003;44:78P.

[63] Tatsumi M, Cohade C, Mourtzikos KA, et al. Initial experience with FDG-PET-CT in the evaluation of breast cancer [abstract]. J Nucl Med 2003;44:394P.

[64] Ciernik F, Dizendorf E, Baumert BG, et al. Radiation treatment planning with an integrated positron emission and computer tomography (PET/CT): A feasibility study. Int J Radiat Oncol Biol Phys 2003;57(3):853–63.

RADIOLOGIC
CLINICS
OF NORTH AMERICA

Radiol Clin N Am 45 (2007) 669–676

ELSEVIER
SAUNDERS

Detection of Bone Metastases in Breast Cancer by Positron Emission Tomography

Holger Schirrmeister, MD

Carcinoma of the breast is the most prevalent cancer in women in the United States and Western Europe, and is commonly associated with metastatic bone disease. The incidence of breast cancer has been increasing in Western Europe and the United States, but the number of deaths resulting from breast cancer has remained relatively stable [1]. This is probably related to more effective treatment strategies and to the detection of disease at early stages.

Although the incidence of bone metastases is as low as 1% to 2% at the time of primary diagnosis [2], bone metastases are found in one third of all patients who have recurrent disease [3]. In a study including 587 patients who died from breast cancer [4], 69% had radiological evidence of skeletal metastases before death. There are two different types of bony metastases—osteolytic and osteoblastic disease—depending on their radiographic appearance. Patients who have breast cancer can have either osteolytic or osteoblastic metastases, or can present with mixed lesions containing both features [5]. Interestingly, patients who have bone metastases only survive 2 to 3 years longer than patients who have visceral involvement. The distribution

of bone metastases is a relevant prognostic factor. Yamashita and colleagues [6,7] reported a significantly longer survival in patients who had bone metastases exclusively to the upper regions of the skeleton than in patients who had metastases to the pelvis and the lower extremities. Furthermore, presence of osteoblastic features in bony metastases was also reported to be associated with prolonged survival [6,7].

It has been estimated that bone metastases become visible on plain radiographs after 30% to 50% of bone mineral loss [8]. Secondary formation of bone also occurs as response to osteolytic destruction; hence, even osteolytic bone metastases can be detected with bone scintigraphy several months before they are apparent on plain radiographs [9,10]. Bone scintigraphy is not perfect in detecting bone metastases, however; comparative studies with MRI revealed significantly more vertebral metastases not detected on conventional planar bone scintigraphy [11,12]. Nevertheless, conventional bone scintigraphy remains the most suitable technique for whole-body screening, because whole-body MRI is currently not practical for routine whole-body surveys, and its sensitivity

This article was previously published in PET Clinics 2006;1:25–32.
Clinic of Nuclear Medicine, University of Kiel, Arnold-Heller Str. 9, Kiel 24105, Germany
E-mail address: hschirrmeister@nuc-med.uni-kiel.de

doi:10.1016/j.rcl.2007.05.007

in detecting extra-vertebral metastases is not yet sufficiently assessed.

Positron emission tomography (PET) is a relatively new imaging technique for noninvasive assessment of several metabolic pathways. During the last decade, this method evolved from a research tool to a standard imaging modality for routine staging of several types of malignant tumors. PET using the glucose analog 2-(fluoro-18)-2-deoxy-D-glucose (FDG) enables detection of primary breast cancer and its metastases on the basis of increased glucose metabolism in neoplastic tissues. Characterization of bone metastases is also possible with F-18 sodium fluoride, which shows ostoblastic bone reaction. The potential of PET with FDG and F-18 fluoride in detecting bone metastases originating from breast cancer is discussed in this article.

F-18 fluoride positron emission tomography

Skeletal uptake of the positron emitter F-18 fluoride is based on the exchange of hydroxyl ions in the hydroxyapatite crystal. Hence, the uptake of F-18 fluoride is an indicator of bone mineralization [13]. F-18 fluoride was introduced into clinical practice by Blau in 1962 [14]. Subsequently, F-18 fluoride was approved by the Food and Drug Administration (FDA) as a radiotracer for bone scintigraphy. One decade later, this radiopharmaceutical was replaced by Tc-99m-labeled polyphosphonates, because conventional gamma cameras performed better in terms of sensitivity and spatial resolution of the 140 keV photons from Tc-99m compared with the 511 keV photons from F-18 fluoride.

In comparing the pharmacokinetics of Tc-99m labeled polyphosphonates and F-18 fluoride, it is important to note that the uptake of F-18 fluoride into bone is approximately twofold higher and the blood clearance is significantly faster compared with technetium labeled polyphosphonates. This leads to an increased bone-to-background ratio for F-18 fluoride. The improved sensitivity and better spatial resolution of modern PET scanners allow performing highly sensitive and specific whole-body screening for bone metastases [15–19]. In a pilot study [16], F-18 fluoride PET revealed two times more bone metastases than bone scintigraphy in patients who had osteolytic disease from thyroid cancer or osteoblastic metastases from prostate cancer. An important finding in this study was that the sensitivity of planar bone scintigraphy was highly variable, depending on the skeletal region. The sensitivity of bone scintigraphy was as low as 20% in the thoracic spine and 40% in the lumbar spine; in contrast, the sensitivity of bone scintigraphy

ranged between 80% and 90% in the skull, thorax, and the extremities. The most probable explanation for these findings is that the detection of vertebral bone metastases was limited by superimposed tracer retention in soft tissue and other parts of the skeleton. This drawback of conventional gamma camera imaging is generally not present with tomographic imaging. Hence, in contrast to conventional bone scintigraphy, the sensitivity of F-18 fluoride PET was independent from the anatomical localization of skeletal lesions [16].

In another prospective study [17], F-18 fluoride PET was performed in 34 patients who had breast cancer and high risk of metastatic bone disease. F-18 fluoride PET revealed more metastases than conventional bone scintigraphy in 11 of 17 patients who had bony metastases. Three patients were true-positive on F-18 fluoride PET, but had no signs of metastatic bone disease on normal bone scintigraphy [Figs. 1, 2]. In another patient who had known metastases, an osteolytic lesion was depicted with F-18 fluoride PET that had been missed

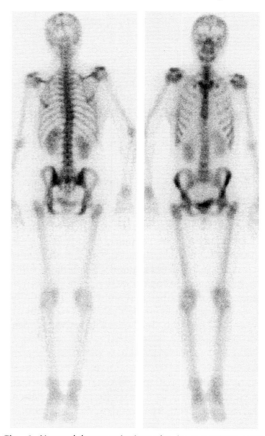

Fig. 1. Normal bone scintigraphy in a patient with breast cancer (pT2,N0). Bone scintigraphy was performed because of increasing serum alkaline phosphatase and calcium levels.

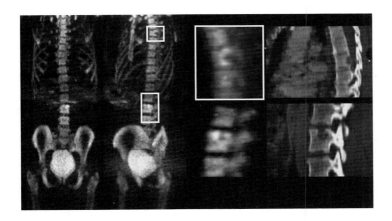

Fig. 2. F-18 fluoride PET of the same patient as presented in Fig. 1. PET imaging was obtained 2 hours after injection of 370 MBq F-18 fluoride. Two osteolytic metastases are present in the thoracic and lumbar spine. Maximum intensity projection images (*left*). Sagittal sections of the thoracic and lumbar spine (*middle*). Corresponding sagittal CT images (*right*).

by bone scintigraphy. Because of the risk for pathologic bone fracture, this metastasis was surgically stabilized. In this highly selected series, clinical management was influenced in 4 out of 34 patients by the results from F-18 fluoride PET.

Along with the twofold higher sensitivity in detecting bone metastases, there is also a twofold higher rate of benign lesions visible on F-18 fluoride PET [16]. In a recent review article [20], it was assumed that this would lead to an increased rate of false-positive results. This assumption, however, is not supported by the current literature, in which the specificity of F-18 fluoride PET was 90% and higher in several studies [16–19].

It is important to note that uptake of F-18 fluoride is not tumor-specific, and that numerous benign lesions are detected by F-18 fluoride PET. Differentiation between benign and malignant bony lesions is not possible by means of quantitative analysis of bone metabolism [21]. Nevertheless, the superior spatial resolution of modern PET scanners allows for exact anatomical localization of lesions and a better differentiation between benign [22] and malignant lesions [23] compared with conventional gamma cameras.

In breast cancer, both osteolytic and osteoblastic bone metastases have been reported to demonstrate focally increased F-18 fluoride uptake [15]. In the

experience of the author's group, osteolytic metastases were often characterized as photopenic lesions surrounded by a rim of increased activity [Fig. 3]. This pattern was observed exclusively in osteolytic metastases and not in benign lesions [23].

Both osteolytic metastases and benign lesions appear as regions with focally increased tracer uptake. Therefore, knowledge of the typical appearance of benign lesions becomes crucial for differentiation between benign lesions and metastases. Arthritis of the articular facets and endplate fractures account for approximately 80% of all benign abnormalities detected with F-18 fluoride PET [22]. These abnormalities have a very characteristic F-18 fluoride uptake pattern [Fig. 4]. Osteophytes are characterized as lesions with variable tracer uptake located at the superior and inferior edges of adjacent endplates, whereas increased F-18 fluoride uptake at adjacent surfaces of intervertebral joints is typical for intervertebral arthritis. On F-18 fluoride PET, lesions neither located at joint surfaces nor showing the typical pattern of endplate fractures, osteophytes, or serial rib fractures are suspicious for metastatic disease [23].

F-18 fluorodeoxyglucose

The glucose analog 2-(fluoro-18)-2-deoxy-D-glucose (FDG) is currently the most commonly used

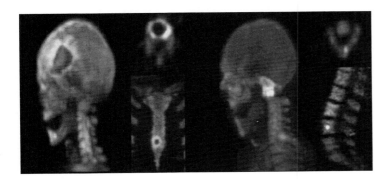

Fig. 3. F-18 fluoride PET. Typical pattern of osteolytic (*left*) and osteoblastic metastases (*right*).

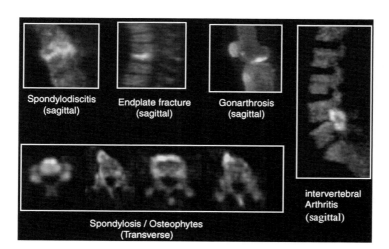

Fig. 4. F-18 fluoride PET. Typical pattern of benign lesions.

radiotracer in oncologic PET imaging. This surrogate marker for glucose metabolism enters the cell via the glucose transporter membrane proteins Glut-1 and Glut-5. FDG is then posphorylated by the enzyme hexokinase. In contrast to glucose, FDG-6-phospate is not a substrate for the glucose-6-phophate isomerase, and is therefore trapped within tumor cells.

Although the exact uptake mechanism of FDG in bone metastases is not yet known, it is assumed that FDG is taken up directly into the tumor tissue of skeletal metastases and not into the surrounding remodeled bone. There are only a few reports addressing the accuracy of FDG-PET for detecting skeletal metastases of breast cancer. This is probably related to the low incidence of bone metastases at initial diagnosis, and the absence of a reliable gold standard.

In a series of 23 breast cancer patients who had metastatic bone disease, Cook and coworkers [24] evaluated FDG-PET in osteoblastic and osteolytic bone metastases by semiquantitative standardized uptake values (SUV). In this series, the FDG uptake was approximately sevenfold higher in osteolytic bone metastases compared with osteoblastic metastases [Figs. 5, 6]. In the entire patient group, FDG-PET detected more bone metastases than bone scintigraphy. Bone scintigraphy, however, was more sensitive in a subgroup of patients who had predominantly osteoblastic disease.

Ohta and colleagues [25] compared the accuracy of conventional bone scintigraphy with FDG-PET in 51 breast cancer patients. In this series, the sensitivity and specificity of FDG-PET were 77.7% and 97.6%, respectively, compared with 77.7% and 80.3% for bone scintigraphy. A similar sensitivity and an even higher specificity were found for FDG-PET compared with bone scintigraphy in a series of 48 patients who had biopsy-proven breast cancer and suspected bone metastases [26]. Comparable results for FDG-PET and bone scintigraphy

were also reported in a series of 24 breast cancer patients by Kao and coworkers [27]. In their study, FDG-PET was less sensitive but significantly more specific than bone scintigraphy.

One limitation of the studies described above is that planer bone scintigraphy was compared with FDG-PET tomographic images. In general, tomographic imaging methods are more sensitive than planar imaging, because lesions are detectable without superposition by other anatomical structures. For example, small lung metastases are seen on CT but frequently not on plain radiographs, and vertebral bone metastases are seen on single photon emission computed tomography (SPECT), CT, or MRI, despite negative planar bone scintigraphy or plain radiographs. Accordingly, Kosuda and colleagues [28] demonstrated a significantly improved sensitivity for detection of bone metastases by SPECT imaging compared with planar bone scintigraphy. The improved sensitivity of bone scintigraphy by using SPECT imaging was also found in a mixed series of 174 patients by Han and coworkers [29]

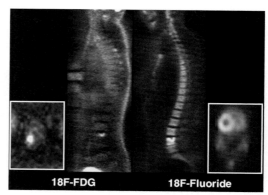

Fig. 5. FDG-PET in a patient with recurrent breast cancer presenting with increased FDG uptake in a small osteolytic metastasis (L-4).

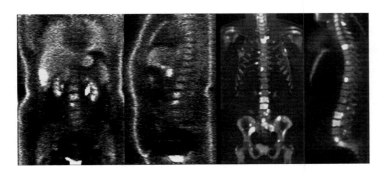

Fig. 6. FDG-PET in a patient with recurrent breast cancer presenting with multiple osteoblastic bone metastases. Intense increased FDG uptake is present in a liver metastasis, whereas the bone metastases show only little FDG uptake.

and in another prospective series of 103 patients who had lung cancer [19].

The first study comparing bone SPECT and FDG-PET was recently published by Uematsu and coworkers [30]. In this study, 15 patients who had known metastatic bone disease were included. CT, MRI, and the subsequent clinical follow-up were used as references. In a lesion-by-lesion analysis, the sensitivity of SPECT was 95%, and only 17% for FDG-PET. The specificity was not statistically significantly different between both imaging methods (SPECT 99%, PET 100%).

The results reported by Cook and colleagues [24] and the studies comparing bone scintigraphy with FDG-PET [25–27,30] indicate that FDG-PET might not be more sensitive than bone scintigraphy but is probably more specific. Because FDG-PET and bone scintigraphy have a different sensitivity for detecting oteoblastic and osteolytic bone metastases, the imaging modalities should be regarded as complementary, but cannot replace each other.

F-18 fluoride positron emission tomography versus F-18 fluorodeoxyglucose-positron emission tomography: which radiotracer should be used in breast cancer?

A prospective comparison of FDG-PET and F-18 fluoride PET in detecting bone metastases from breast cancer has not yet been published. A recent study [19] evaluated the accuracy and cost-effectiveness of F-18 fluoride PET in 103 patients who had initial diagnosis of lung cancer. In this study, FDG-PET was performed for whole-body staging in 41 patients, 10 of whom had bone metastases. One of these patients had disseminated bone metastases, but was negative on FDG-PET. Furthermore, the number of bone metastases was underestimated in an additional 4 patients. The results of this study are in line with the results of the study reported by Uesuda and coworkers [30], who compared bone SPECT and FDG-PET. Both studies indicated a significantly better sensitivity by using bone-specific radiotracers in combination with tomographic imaging (SPECT or PET). An interesting finding of that study was that 2 patients who had highly suspicious vertebral metastases on MRI were negative on F-18 fluoride PET. Skeletal metastases were ruled out by clinical follow-up in 1 patient and by biopsy in the other patient. F-18 fluoride PET might therefore become the first imaging method that is sensitive and specific enough for confirmation of suspicious lesions that are seen on MRI, but are negative on currently available conventional imaging methods.

One important advantage of FDG over F-18 fluoride is that the FDG uptake is not limited to bone metabolism. Several studies have shown that

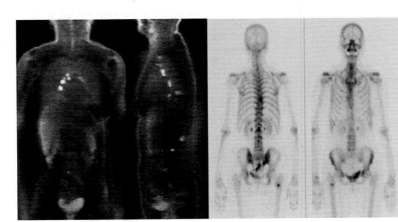

Fig. 7. FDG-PET (*left*) and bone scintigraphy (*right*) was performed for restaging in a patient with recurrent breast cancer. FDG-PET shows multiple lymph node metastases but fewer bone metastases compared with bone scintigraphy.

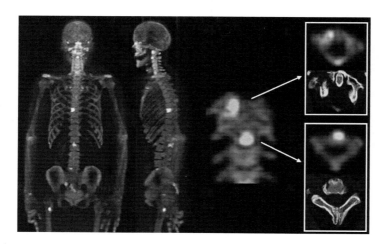

Fig. 8. F-18 fluoride PET of the same patient as presented in Fig. 7. F-18 fluoride PET was performed because the patient complained of neck stiffness and a suspicious lesion was seen on MRI in the second cervical vertebral body. The F-18 fluoride PET scan confirms the bone metastasis by intense increased bone metabolism and reveals an additional, previously unsuspected, bone metastasis in first cervical vertebral body (*arrows*).

FDG-PET reliably detects primary tumors [31–36], and is currently the most sensitive imaging technique for noninvasive assessment of axillary lymph nodes and visceral metastases. Furthermore, Eubank and colleagues [37] have shown that FDG-PET is accurate in evaluating the internal lymph nodes. FDG PET was superior to conventional imaging and as sensitive as MRI in the differentiation between unifocal and multifocal disease [38]. In a series of 117 patients who had suspected breast cancer [36], whole-body FDG-PET was as accurate as the currently employed imaging methods in identification of the primary tumor, and significantly more accurate in the detection of lymph node and distant metastases. In that series, only 2 patients had bone metastases. Both were true-positive on both bone scintigraphy and FDG-PET. Because of the low incidence of bone metastases, a potentially lower sensitivity in detecting osteoblastic bone metastases with FDG-PET seems less relevant at initial staging.

Regarding the specificity in evaluation of the skeleton, there are some rare benign bone tumors and inflammatory lesions that demonstrate increased FDG uptake. In contrast, the uptake of F-18 fluoride is not limited to malignant bone lesions. In turn, F-18 PET fluoride requires specific experience with this method. This limitation might be overcome by using coregistered PET and CT images (PET/CT). Recently Even-Sapir and coworkers [39] found a significantly higher accuracy of F-18 fluoride PET/CT compared with F-18 fluoride PET in a mixed series of 44 cancer patients.

Summary

FDG-PET might be less sensitive than F-18 fluoride PET in detecting bone metastases from breast cancer, but FDG-PET allows accurate assessment of the primary tumor, lymph nodes, and visceral metastases in one single imaging study. The uptake of FDG is more specific for malignant lesions than bone metabolic radiotracers. Hence, FDG-PET in combination with bone scintigraphy might become the standard of care for staging and restaging of the skeleton in breast cancer. F-18 fluoride PET is currently the most sensitive whole-body imaging modality for bone metastases, but is associated with a significant learning curve. In breast cancer, the the use of F-18 fluoride PET should be based on individual cases [Figs. 7, 8] depending on the expected change of therapy management.

References

[1] Newcomb PA, Lantz PM. Recent trends in breast cancer incidence, mortality, and mammography. Breast Cancer Res Treat 1993;28(2):97–106.

[2] Perez DJ, Powles TJ, Milan J, et al. Detection of breast carcinoma metastases in bone: relative merits of x-rays and skeletal scintigraphy in breast cancer. Lancet 1983;10;2(8350):613–6.

[3] Kunkler IH, Merrick MV. The value of non-staging skeletal scintigraphy. Clin Radiol 1986; 37(6):561–2.

[4] Coleman RE, Rubens RD. the clinical course of bone metastases from breast cancer. Br J Cancer 1987;55:61–6.

[5] Hortobagyi GN. Bone metastases in breast cancer patients. Semin Oncol 1991;18(Suppl 5):11–5.

[6] Yamashita K, Koyama H, Inaji H. Prognostic significance of bone metastasis from breast cancer. Clin Orthop 1995;312:89–94.

[7] Yamashita K, Ueda T, Komatsubara Y, et al. Breast cancer with bone-only metastases. Visceral metastases-free rate in relation to anatomic distribution of bone metastases. Cancer 1991;68(3): 634–7.

[8] Bachman AS, Sproul EE. Correlation of radiographic and autopsy findings in suspected

metastases in the spine. Bull N Y Acad Med 1940; 44:169–75.

[9] Silberstein ER, Saenger EL, Tofe AJ, et al. Imaging of bone metastases with ^{99m}Tc-Sn-HEDP (diphosphonate), ^{18}F and skeletal radiography. Radiology 1973;107:551–5.

[10] Green D, Jeremy R, Towson J, et al. The role of fluorine 18 scanning in the detection of skeletal metastases in early breast cancer. Aust N Z J Surg 1973;43:251–4.

[11] Frank JA, Ling A, Patronas NJ, et al. Detection of malignant bone tumors: MR imaging vs scintigraphy. AJR Am J Roentgenol 1990;155:1043–8.

[12] Gosfield E, Alavi A, Kneeland B. Comparison of radionuclide bone scans and magnetic resonance imaging in detecting spinal metastases. J Nucl Med 1993;34:2191–8.

[13] Hawkins RA, Choi Y, Huang SC, et al. Evaluation of skeletal kinetics of fluorine 18-fluoride ion with PET. J Nucl Med 1992;33:633–64.

[14] Blau M, Nagler W, Bender MA. Fluorine-18 a new isotope for bone scanning. J Nucl Med 1962;3:332–4.

[15] Petren-Mallmin M, Andreasson I, Ljunggren O, et al. Skeletal metastases from breast cancer: uptake of F-18 fluoride measured with positron emission tomography in correlation with CT. Skeletal Radiol 1998;27(2):72–6.

[16] Schirrmeister H, Guhlmann CA, Elsner K, et al. Planar bone imaging vs. 18F-PET in patients with cancer of the prostate, thyroid and lung. J Nucl Med 1999;40(10):1623–9.

[17] Schirrmeister H, Guhlmann CA, Kotzerke J, et al. Early detection and accurate description of extent of metastatic bone disease in breast cancer with 18F-fluoride ion and positron emission tomograpy. J Clin Onol 1999;17(8):2381–9.

[18] Schirrmeister H, Glatting G, Hetzel J, et al. Prospective evaluation of the clinical value of planar bone scans, SPECT and F-18 labelled NaF PET in newly diagnosed lung cancer. J Nucl Med 2001; 42(12):1800–4.

[19] Hetzel M, Arslandemir C, König HH, et al. F-18 NaF PET for detection of bone metastases in lung cancer. Accuracy, cost-effectiveness, and impact on patient management. J Bone Miner Res 2003;18(12):2206–14.

[20] Buscombe JR, Holloway B, Roche N, et al. Position of nuclear medicine modalities in the diagnostic work-up of breast cancer. Q J Nucl Med Mol Imaging 2004;48(2):109–18.

[21] Hoh CK, Hawkins RA, Dahlbom M, et al. Whole body skeletal imaging with 18F fluoride ion and PET. J Comput Assist Tomogr 1993;17(1):34–41.

[22] Schirrmeister H, Diederichs CG, Rentschler M, et al. Die Positronenemissionstomographie des Skelettsystems mit ^{18}FNa: Häufigkeit, Befundmuster und Verteilung benigner Veränderungen [Positron-emission tomography of the skeletal system using 18FNa: the incidence, pattern of the findings and distribution of benign changes]. Fortschr Röntgenstr 1998;169(3):310–4 [in German].

[23] Schirrmeister H, Guhlmann CA, Elsner K, et al. Die Positronenemissionstomographie des Skelettsystems mit ^{18}FNa: Häufigkeit, Befundmuster und Verteilung von Skelettmetastasen [Positron emission tomography of the skeletal system using 18FNa: frequency, distribution and appearance of skeletal metastases]. Rontgenpraxis 1999;52(1):19–25 [in German].

[24] Cook GJ, Houston S, Rubens R, et al. Detection of bone metastases in breast cancer by 18FDG PET: differing metabolic activity in osteoblastic and osteolytic lesions. J Clin Oncol 1998; 16(10):3375–9.

[25] Ohta M, Tokuda Y, Suzuki Y, et al. Whole body PET for the evaluation of bony metastases in patients with breast cancer: comparison with 99mTc-MDP bone scintigraphy. Nucl Med Commun 2001;22(8):875–9.

[26] Yang SN, Liang JA, Lin FJ, et al. Comparing whole body 18F-2-deoxyglucose positron emission tomography and technetium-99m methylene diphophonate bone scan to detect bone metastases in patients with breast cancer. J Cancer Res Clin Oncol 2002;128(6): 325–8.

[27] Kao CH, Hsieh JF, Tsai SC, et al. Comparison and discrepancy of 18F-deoxyglucose-positron emission tomography and Tc-99m MDP bone scan to detect bone metastases. Anticancer Res 2000; 20(3B):2189–92.

[28] Kosuda S, Kaji T, Yokoyama H, et al. Does bone SPECT actually have lower sensitivity for detecting vertebral metastasis than MRI? J Nucl Med 1996;37(6):975–8.

[29] Han LJ, Au-Yong TK, Tong WC, et al. Comparison of bone single-photon emission tomography and planar imaging in the detection of vertebral metastases in patients with back pain. Eur J Nucl Med 1998;25(6):635–8.

[30] Uematsu T, Yuen S, Yukisawa S, et al. Comparison of FDG PET and SPECT for detection of bone metastases in breast cancer. AJR Am J Roentgenol 2005;184(4):1266–73.

[31] Adler LP, Crowe JP, Al-Kaisi NK, et al. Evaluation of breast masses and axillary lymph nodes with F-18 2-deoxy-3-fluoro-D-glucose. Radiology 1993;187(3):743–50.

[32] Avril N, Dose J, Jänicke F, et al. Assessment of axillary lymph node involvment in breast cancer patients with positron emission tomography using radiolabeled 2-(fluorine-18)-deoxy-2-fluoro-D-glucose. J Natl Cancer Inst 1996;88(17): 1204–9.

[33] Crippa F, Agresti R, Seregni E, et al. Prospective evaluation of fluorine-18-FDG PET in presurgical staging of the axilla in breast cancer. J Nucl Med 1998;39(1):4–8.

[34] Moon DH, Maddahi J, Silverman DHS, et al. Accuracy of whole-body fluorine-18 FDG PET for the detection of recurrent or metastatic breast carcinoma. J Nucl Med 1998;39(3): 431–5.

[35] Eubank WB, Mankoff DA, Vesselle HJ, et al. Detection of locoregional and distant recurrences in breast cancer patients by using FDG PET. Radiographics 2002;22(1):5–17.

[36] Schirrmeister H, Kuhn T, Guhlmann A, et al. Fluorine-18 2-deoxy-2-fluoro-D-glucose PET in the preoperative staging of breast cancer: comparison with the standard staging procedures. Eur J Nucl Med 2001;28(3):351–8.

[37] Eubank WB, Mankoff DA, Takasugi J, et al. 18fluorodeoxyglucose positron emission tomography to detect mediastinal or internal mammary metastases in breast cancer. J Clin Oncol 2001; 19(15):3516–23.

[38] Rieber A, Schirrmeister H, Gabelmann A, et al. Pre-operative staging of invasive breast cancer with MR mammography and/or PET: boon or bunk? Br J Radiol 2002;75(898): 789–98.

[39] Even-Sapir E, Metser U, Flusser G, et al. Assessment of malignant skeletal disease: initial experience with 18F-fluoride PET/CT and comparison between 18F-fluoride PET and 18F-fluoride PET/CT. J Nucl Med 2004;45(2):272–8.

RADIOLOGIC
CLINICS
OF NORTH AMERICA

Radiol Clin N Am 45 (2007) 677–688

ELSEVIER
SAUNDERS

Normal and Abnormal Patterns of 18F-Fluorodeoxyglucose PET/CT in Lymphoma

Rachel Bar-Shalom, MD[a,b,*]

- 18F-fluorodeoxyglucose PET/CT in pretherapy assessment of lymphoma
- 18F-fluorodeoxyglucose PET/CT in posttherapy assessment of lymphoma
- 18F-fluorodeoxyglucose PET/CT regional anatomy for assessment of lymphoma
- Summary
- References

Lymphoma has an overall cure rate of up to 80%, which is achieved by the use of multiple combined therapeutic modalities. The high rate of response to treatment and prolonged survival, along with the wide range of therapeutic options and their potential side effects, demand accurate pretherapy assessment of the extent of disease, timely estimation of the individual patient's chemosensitivity, and early detection of relapse.

Imaging plays an important role in the noninvasive assessment of patients with lymphoma, with its main purpose being to provide the means for assessment of risk and response-adapted therapy [1,2]. Although CT is currently the main modality for morphologic assessment of lymphoma, PET using 18F-fluorodeoxyglucose (FDG) has taken the place of gallium-67 scintigraphy as the modality of choice for functional and metabolic imaging of these patients. FDG-PET has been shown to be superior to CT in various indications [3–7]. FDG-PET is of value for the initial staging of lymphoma [8–13], for monitoring the response to various therapeutic protocols

[14–19], for prognostic stratification, and for detection of relapse during follow-up [16–18,20–23].

The limitations of CT and FDG-PET in the assessment of lymphoma have been documented as well. They stem mainly from different technique-related characteristics and may be overcome by the complementary use of both modalities [8–10,13]. Limitations of CT in the assessment of lymphoma result from the inaccuracy of size criteria or attenuation-related tissue properties for the diagnosis of lymphoma, which leads to the inability of CT to identify disease in nodes or organs of normal size and texture or to differentiate between residual mass and viable lymphoma after treatment [1,24].

Although FDG-PET has been reported to have high sensitivity and specificity for the detection of lymphoma, this modality also has limitations related to several factors, including the inherent difficulties in clear topographic orientation of PET findings in high target-to-background images, the nonspecific FDG uptake in physiologic or non-lymphomatous processes, and, to a lesser extent,

This article was previously published in PET Clinics 2006;1:231–42.
[a] Division of Positron Emission Tomography, Department of Nuclear Medicine, Rambam Health Care Campus, Haifa, 35254 Israel
[b] B. Rapaport School of Medicine, Israel Institute of Technology-Technion, Haifa, Israel
* Department of Nuclear Medicine, Rambam Health Care Campus, Haifa, 35254 Israel.
E-mail address: r_bar_shalom@rambam.health.gov.il

doi:10.1016/j.rcl.2007.05.006

the variability in FDG avidity of several histologic lymphoma types [13,19,23,25–27].

PET/CT systems provide accurate coregistration of sequential near-simultaneous acquisition of PET and CT. One of the main advantages of PET/CT is the accurate localization of sites of increased FDG uptake to anatomic structures defined by CT [28]. This precise localization is important for the differentiation between foci of physiologic tracer uptake and lymphoma involvement, especially when in close proximity. Accurate localization of malignant sites to a specific organ or node may be clinically important not only for the diagnosis of lymphoma but for the definition of disease extent as well as for directing the further diagnostic and therapeutic approach. Fused PET/CT data may lead to retrospective detection of lymphoma sites previously overlooked on either PET or CT, such as lesions with mild FDG uptake, lesions located within regions of complex anatomy, or lesions showing extensive morphologic abnormalities on CT [7,28–35].

Variable normal and abnormal patterns of FDG uptake in patients with lymphoma at various time points during the course of disease have been discerned with the use of PET/CT and are presented in the following review. Recognition and characterization of these patterns are important for accurate interpretation of findings and, at times, for further clinical management.

¹⁸F-fluorodeoxyglucose PET/CT in pretherapy assessment of lymphoma

At initial staging, FDG-PET has been shown to be more accurate than CT, with a reported sensitivity and specificity greater than 90% [10,13,36,37]. The detection of additional nodal and extranodal sites as well as exclusion of disease suspected on CT has been reported to change the staging of disease in 14% to 59% of patients with lymphoma [8,11,32,38–41]. PET/CT can also have incremental value with respect to several aspects of disease staging. Diagnosis of all sites of lymphoma involvement, above and below the diaphragm, is of the utmost clinical importance for accurate staging. PET/CT can delineate the position of a specific site as located below or above the diaphragm, such as the differentiation of a retrocrural node from an abdominal node or of supradiaphragmatic lymph nodes from peritoneal lymph nodes (Fig. 1).

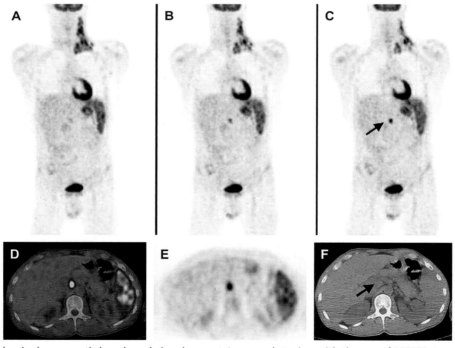

Fig. 1. Abdominal para-aortic lymph node involvement. Improved staging with the use of PET/CT. A patient with lymphoma presented with multiple disease sites, including the left cervical and supraclavicular region and the spleen, corresponding to findings seen on CT, and thus defined as stage II$_S$ disease. (*A, B, C*) Coronal PET images show intense uptake in the known supradiaphragmatic sites and in the enlarged spleen. In addition, there is a focus of abnormal FDG uptake in the upper abdomen (*arrow*). PET/CT (*D*) localizes the focal abdominal uptake seen on PET (*E*) within an abdominal right para-aortic lymph node only retrospectively recognized on CT (*F*), upstaging the disease to stage III.

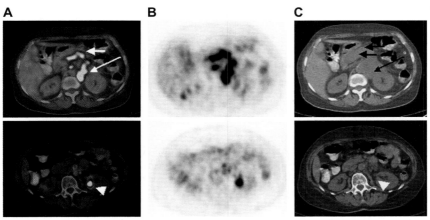

Fig. 2. Detection of extranodal lymphoma on PET/CT. PET/CT (*A*) enables the accurate characterization of PET findings (*B*), differentiating between nodal retroperitoneal left para-aortic adenopathy (*long arrows*) and extranodal involvement in the body of the pancreas (*short arrows*) and the left kidney (*arrowheads*), as seen on CT (*C*).

Although at the level of the diaphragm and upper abdominal region, PET/CT images may be prone to misregistration because of respiratory motion, different methods have been developed to improve image registration, such as breath-hold CT acquisition at normal expiration or respiratory gating [8,35,42,43].

The detection of extranodal lymphoma involvement can affect disease staging and may be of value for guiding further diagnostic investigations and follow-up after treatment. PET has been reported as having a higher accuracy for identification of extranodal disease as compared with CT [30,37]. PET/CT can be of additional value in the assessment of extranodal disease by differentiating it from tracer activity in regions of relative abundant physiologic FDG uptake, such as the abdomen and pelvis, or from adjacent lymph node involvement (Fig. 2). Fused images may also pinpoint a previously missed extranodal site erroneously considered to represent lymphomatous adenopathy in regions of complicated anatomy, such as the head and neck (Fig. 3) [29,30,34,35].

Although it is still unclear what percentage of lymphomas are non-FDG avid and whether baseline pretherapy studies are needed for accurate posttreatment follow-up with PET, some reports indicate lower FDG avidity for low-grade non-

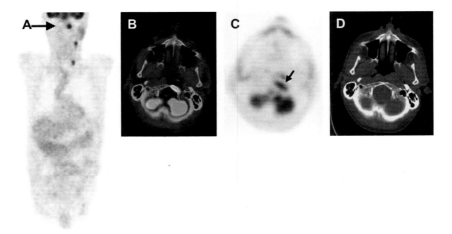

Fig. 3. Diagnosis of lymphoma sites in complicated anatomic regions by PET/CT. (*A*) Several foci of abnormal FDG uptake in the head and neck region are seen on the coronal PET image in the left cervical region and possibly in the left pharynx (*arrow*). PET/CT (*B*) precisely localizes this PET focus (*arrow, C*) to its corresponding anatomic location on CT (*D*), defining skeletal involvement of lymphoma of the occipital bone in the left anterior margin of the foramen magnum.

Hodgkin's lymphoma (NHL), particularly periph- eral T-cell, mucosa-associated lymphoid tissue (MALT), and small lymphocytic subtypes [5,9,25,44]. PET/CT can enable the recognition of low-intensity FDG uptake within regions of lymph- adenopathy or other pathologic lesions on CT that might be otherwise ignored or mistaken for physio- logic tracer activity in the bowel, urinary tract, ves- sels, or muscles [31]. PET/CT may be also useful for the detection of small lesions that may be missed on PET or CT, such as those located in the base of the lungs or in peripheral sites, as is the case with lymphoma of the skin [45]. Retrospective detection of foci of even mild tracer uptake on PET or the recognition of previously ignored small lesions on CT has been induced by coregistration of both modalities (Fig. 4) [28].

18F-fluorodeoxyglucose PET/CT in posttherapy assessment of lymphoma

With appropriate therapy, the chances for cure are high, even in cases of recurrent lymphoma. Accurate assessment of the response to therapy and follow-up of patients who have achieved a com- plete response, with the purpose of early diagnosis of relapse, are thus clinically significant for improv- ing patient outcome.

Precise assessment of disease status during therapy and after its completion may be problem- atic with CT in the presence of a residual mass or of treatment-related structural abnormalities.

Although residual masses are frequent after therapy and have been encountered in up to 60% of pa- tients with lymphoma, viable residual lymphoma is found in only 18% of these morphologic abnor- malities [24]. Early detection of residual or recur- rent lymphoma within residual masses, while the tumor load is still small, enables the administration of an alternative potentially more effective therapy, with potentially higher chances for success. Con- versely, exclusion of disease in areas of nonviable structural abnormalities can avoid further futile in- vestigations or treatment associated with patient distress, high morbidity, and unnecessary cost.

FDG-PET is a valuable tool for the evaluation of response to therapy early during therapy as well as after its completion [14–17,19,20]. As with initial staging, PET/CT can improve interpretation of FDG-PET by optimized localization and character- ization of suspicious FDG foci after therapy, leading to an accurate assessment of their clinical signifi- cance. Specific difficulties encountered in the assess- ment of patients with lymphoma during and after treatment can be resolved with the use of PET/CT [26,27].

The precise PET definition of response to treat- ment has not been standardized yet. Some consider total disappearance of abnormal tracer uptake as a prerequisite to define complete remission, whereas others advocate assessment of changes in the number or intensity of FDG foci [14,15,17, 20,46]. PET/CT can be useful for better characteri- zation of sites with low-intensity FDG uptake, thus

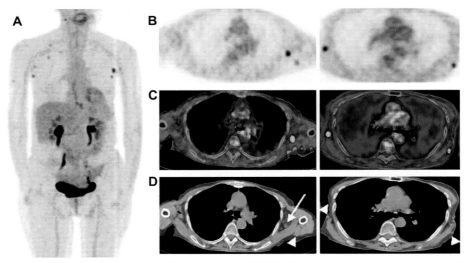

Fig. 4. Detection of small peripheral lymphoma sites by PET/CT. (*A*) Maximum intensity projection (MIP) PET image of this patient with an upper trunk skin lesion diagnosed as NHL shows multiple foci of FDG uptake of variable intensity in the axillary region bilaterally. PET findings (*B*) are localized and characterized by PET/CT (*C*) as sites of disease in the peripheral skin lesions (*arrowheads*) and left axillary lymph node (*long arrow*) seen on CT (*D*).

confirming or excluding disease in these foci. The detection of minimal residual disease during therapy or recurrence in regions of faint FDG uptake may be important for therapeutic decisions concerning the initiation or modification of therapy.

FDG-PET may provide accurate information on the presence of viable lymphoma within residual masses seen on CT after treatment [20–23]. The precise spatial localization of abnormal tracer uptake within residual morphologic changes or in a specific anatomic structure, even in the absence of overt structural pathologic findings, may be difficult but of major clinical significance. PET/CT can direct further invasive procedures for tissue confirmation of FDG-avid areas within large heterogeneous residual masses seen on CT and guide further exploration of normal-sized PET-positive lymph nodes and other lesions with minimal structural changes. PET/CT can also allow the recognition of subtle anatomic abnormalities on CT that were ignored before coregistration with PET findings (Fig. 5). PET/CT data may be used to guide radiotherapy planning to include viable residual or recurrent malignant tissue and to prevent toxic radiation effect in adjacent nonviable or healthy tissues [7,13,34,47].

In patients with low-grade NHL, an increase in the intensity of FDG activity in sites of disease that have previously shown a low degree of uptake was suggested as an indicator for possible histologic transformation [34,48]. PET/CT can be used to direct biopsy to such nodes or to specific areas within the same lymph node to enable tissue confirmation of this potential transformation with significant prognostic and therapeutic implications.

Limitations of FDG-PET in monitoring the response to treatment of lymphoma are related mainly to the inherent nonspecific FDG uptake in inflammatory or infectious processes, which is encountered more frequently with therapy, and to the limited spatial resolution of this imaging modality, which may impair the detection of low residual or recurrent tumor burden [5,26,27,34,49]. Several physiologic or benign FDG uptake patterns, some of them discerned only after the introduction of PET/CT imaging, need to be recognized, especially after completion of therapy, so as to avoid misinterpretation and false-positive reports.

Increased FDG uptake in the thymus, particularly that related to rebound thymic hyperplasia after treatment, has been described in children and young adults and may occur months after completing therapy [50]. The appearance of typical bilobar, arrow-shaped, anterior mediastinal FDG uptake at the characteristic timing in relation to therapy can be highly suggestive for this benign entity (Fig. 6). Differentiation from mediastinal lymphomatous involvement may be difficult at times, however. The precise localization of FDG-avid sites to the anatomic structure corresponding to the thymus on CT, sometimes in an unusual location, may be useful and may exclude disease or direct further investigations, such as ultrasound (US), MRI, or invasive diagnostic procedures when indicated.

A benign pattern of increased FDG uptake in metabolically active brown fat, which is often seen in patients with lymphoma after treatment, has been recognized only after the use of PET/CT [51,52]. This uptake pattern, considered initially as representing increased FDG uptake in tense cervical muscles on PET alone, can be seen in the supraclavicular and shoulder girdle regions, around large vessels in the mediastinum, and in multiple infradiaphragmatic sites (eg, paracolic and perirenal regions). FDG uptake in brown fat may be asymmetric, focal, and highly intense. It may also coexist with lymphomatous adenopathy. Without the use of PET/CT, such uptake cannot be characterized as benign and differentiated from adjacent sites of disease involvement (Fig. 7).

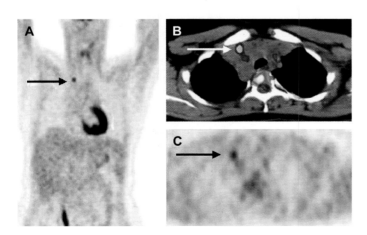

Fig. 5. Detection of recurrent lymphoma within a residual mass by PET/CT. (*A*) Coronal PET image performed during follow-up of a patient with mediastinal HD shows a small focus of abnormal uptake in the upper mediastinal region (*arrow*). (*B*) PET/CT pinpoints the focal uptake seen on PET (*C*) to a small region in the right anterior aspect of a large mediastinal residual mass seen on CT (*arrow*). A PET/CT-guided biopsy confirmed the presence of recurrent mediastinal lymphoma.

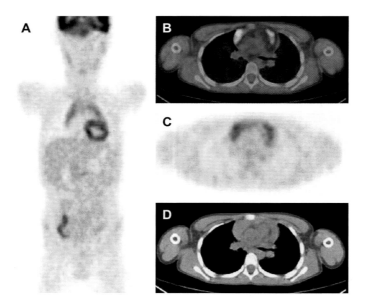

Fig. 6. Characterization of FDG uptake in a hyperplastic thymus by PET/CT. Bilobar arrow-shaped uptake is seen in the mediastinum on the coronal PET image (A) of an 11-year-old patient with lymphoma who was assessed 18 months after completing chemotherapy. PET/CT (B) localizes the uptake seen on PET (C) in a hyperplastic thymus seen on CT (D).

Inflammation poses a diagnostic challenge for defining FDG-avid sites in patients with lymphoma, before and after therapy, because it can mimic residual or recurrent disease [26,27,49]. The attention to detailed patient history and clinical data, recognition of characteristic uptake patterns, and coregistration of PET with CT data can be helpful, although not always conclusive, for accurate diagnosis. Scar tissue in regions of prior invasive diagnostic procedures, insertion of intravenous lines for administration of therapy, or interventional procedures not related to lymphoma may demonstrate intense FDG uptake, usually subsiding in intensity with time. Localization of such uptake along structural changes on CT can indicate its benign nature. Postradiation inflammation can be seen even months after radiotherapy. Chemotherapy may induce lung toxicity with an associated

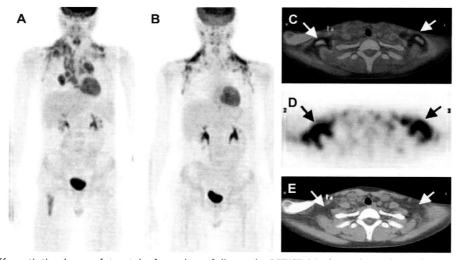

Fig. 7. Differentiating brown fat uptake from sites of disease by PET/CT. Maximum intensity projection (MIP) PET image (A) at the initial staging of a child with Hodgkin's disease diagnosed by a biopsy of a right cervical lymph node demonstrates multiple sites of disease in the neck bilaterally, in the mediastinum, and in the right femur. A repeat MIP PET image (B) of the same patient after therapy shows multiple foci of increased uptake in the cervical and supraclavicular region bilaterally. Persistent disease cannot be excluded in these areas. PET/CT (C) localizes the FDG uptake (arrows) seen on PET (D) to normal fatty tissue seen on CT in these regions (E), characterizing it as benign brown fat uptake, excluding disease, and defining complete remission.

inflammatory reaction. Variable patterns of FDG uptake can be seen on PET in relation to these processes. Diffusely increased and well-demarcated lung uptake can be recognized on PET/CT within regions of postradiation pneumonitis for 4 to 6 months after radiotherapy [26,27]. A relative decrease in skeletal FDG uptake in regions of radiation-induced fibrosis, such as in the pelvis or spine, can create an asymmetric uptake pattern that may be misleading unless correlated with the clinical history and morphologic data.

Inflammatory processes of various infectious or granulomatous etiologies may affect patients with lymphoma. FDG uptake in nodal or extranodal sites involved in these benign processes has been previously described, such as in soft tissue abscesses, herpes zoster, sarcoidosis, and transforming germinal centers [26,27]. PET/CT, correlated with clinical data, can suggest the benign nature of such findings when they are located in specific structural abnormalities. PET/CT can also be used to direct diagnostic biopsy, which may sometimes be the only way to exclude lymphoma in these sites.

¹⁸F-fluorodeoxyglucose PET/CT regional anatomy for assessment of lymphoma

One of the significant advantages of PET in the assessment of lymphoma, which is a multifocal disease, is the ability to screen the whole body. Difficulties in PET interpretation in various anatomic regions can be solved by the use of PET/CT.

In the region of the head and neck, the presence of disease involvement in various structures or organs, such as the retrobulbar or orbital region, pharynx, thyroid, and cervical spine, needs to be defined and differentiated from regional cervical adenopathy. PET/CT can provide this accurate localization of sites of lymphoma. Physiologic tracer activity in the area of the head and neck can be related to muscular activity or to benign salivary or lacrimal gland uptake [26,27]. Whereas mild symmetric uptake in salivary glands can usually be characterized as physiologic or attributable to inflammatory or obstructive processes, prior surgery or radiotherapy may result in a focal, intense, asymmetric uptake, which can be difficult to differentiate from disease in neighboring regional lymph nodes [31,53]. PET/CT can exclude or confirm the presence of lymphoma in equivocal foci of increased FDG uptake.

The precise localization of PET findings in the thorax, a common site of lymphoma involvement, may be important for further patient management at staging and during follow-up. The differentiation between hilar and mediastinal nodal disease can affect the staging of lymphoma. This is also true for the differentiation between nodal mediastinal disease and lung involvement or between axillary and peripheral lung or rib lesions [31]. As mentioned previously, recognizing stage IV disease has potential clinical implications for further diagnostic and therapeutic decisions.

The abdomen and pelvis may be especially challenging for the interpretation of FDG-PET because of the physiologic uptake in multiple abdominal organs and the proximity of various sites of potential lymphoma involvement. Assessment of uptake foci in adjacent structures in the abdomen and pelvis can be facilitated by the use of fused images. PET/CT can define liver or spleen involvement versus adjacent nodal disease, peritoneal versus bowel disease, or physiologic activity as well as differentiating retroperitoneal disease from adjacent physiologic ureteral or adrenal uptake (Fig. 8) [31,35,54]. PET/CT localization of FDG uptake to uncommon sites of lymphoma involvement, such as the testis, prostate, ovary, or uterine cervix, can provide a precise diagnosis of the unsuspected extent of disease and guide further invasive investigations when indicated. Variable patterns of FDG biodistribution in the abdomen and pelvis can be identified on PET/CT, such as the identification of tracer uptake in a bowel loop within an inguinal hernia, in a bladder diverticulum, or in vascular calcifications (Fig. 9) [55,56]. The physiologic variability of FDG uptake in the endometrium and ovaries during the different phases of the menstrual cycle has been characterized by PET/CT [57]. Physiologically increased uptake can be seen in premenopausal women in ovarian follicles as well as in the endometrium during ovulation and menstruation and should be differentiated from regional lymph node or visceral lymphoma involvement in this region, whereas such uptake should be suspicious for the presence of active disease when seen in postmenopausal women [35,57].

Although showing a linear diffuse pattern of mild intensity activity as a rule, physiologic bowel and gastric uptake of FDG may be focal and intense and may mimic lymphoma or obscure adjacent nodal or peritoneal disease. Conversely, mild FDG uptake related to the presence of lymphoma in these organs may be overlooked unless localized to morphologic abnormalities by PET/CT [26,27, 31,35]. Fused images can also distinguish physiologic bowel or gastric uptake from adjacent regional mesenteric or peritoneal lymph node involvement. The mere localization of FDG uptake within the gastrointestinal tract (GIT) by PET/CT cannot always exclude the presence of disease. Incidental foci of FDG uptake in the GIT have been diagnosed as malignant or premalignant in approximately 60% of patients with cancer [58]. The use of oral

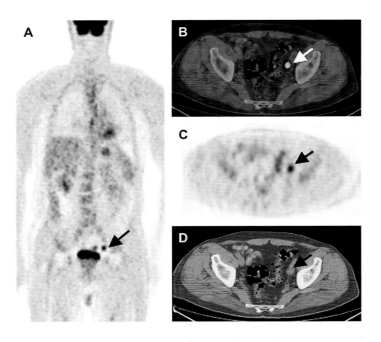

Fig. 8. Left pelvic increased FDG uptake. PET/CT is used for the differential diagnosis between a malignant and benign etiology. (*A*) Coronal PET image demonstrates focally increased FDG uptake in the left pelvic region (*arrow*), which can represent malignant adenopathy or physiologic focal ureteral activity. PET/CT (*B*) characterizes the focus seen on PET (*C*) as malignant by its localization to a left external iliac lymph node (*arrows*) seen on CT (*D*).

and intravenous contrast during CT acquisition on PET/CT provides good intestinal and vascular enhancement without compromising PET quality [59]. Better delineation of intestinal structures and improved differentiation between vascular and adjacent soft tissue structures can further increase the diagnostic power of PET/CT [35].

Whole-body screening provided by FDG-PET is advantageous for assessing the presence of lymphomatous involvement in the musculoskeletal system and in sites located in peripheral regions that are not routinely assessed by conventional morphologic imaging modalities [26,60]. PET/CT can define bone involvement adjacent to disease in the soft tissues, exclude skeletal disease by differentiating vertebral from prevertebral nodal involvement, and identify neural plexus invasion of lymphoma at the region of the neural foramen

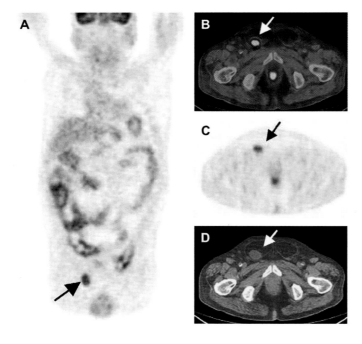

Fig. 9. Defining physiologic uptake in aberrant anatomy in the pelvis by PET/CT. (*A*) Coronal PET image of a patient with aggressive NHL assessed after treatment demonstrates focally intense uptake in the right inguinal region (*arrow*), raising the suspicion of recurrent nodal disease. PET/CT image (*B*) localizes the uptake (*arrows*) seen on PET (*C*) within a bladder herniation into the right groin seen on CT (*D*), characterizing it as physiologic urine activity in an aberrant location.

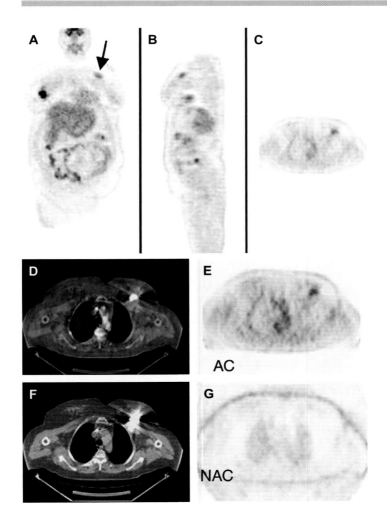

Fig. 10. Artifactual FDG uptake. PET/CT is used for exclusion of disease in sites with metal devices. (*A–C*) PET images of this patient with breast lymphoma before treatment show intense focal uptake in the known right breast lesion. Another focus is seen in the left chest region (*arrow*), possibly representing an additional site of lymphoma. PET/CT (*D*) localizes the uptake in the left chest seen on the attenuation-corrected (AC) PET scan (*E*) to a pacemaker seen on the CT scan (*F*). The increased FDG uptake is not seen on the non–attenuation-corrected (NAC) PET image (*G*), indicating that this is an attenuation correction–related artifact in the region of a metal implant.

AC

NAC

and within the epidural space [61]. Skeletal lesions unrelated to lymphoma, such as degenerative changes in the spine, osteophytes, or fractures, can be differentiated from sites of skeletal lymphoma based on the diagnosis of bone lesions on the CT component of the PET/CT study.

Precise localization of suspicious peripheral sites of tracer uptake to skin folds; along a specific muscle group; or to a region of prior surgery, a central line, or a pacemaker can exclude the presence of lymphomatous involvement in these regions. The non–attenuation-corrected images always have to be reviewed along with the fused data so as to exclude attenuation correction–related artifacts in regions with known metal devices (Fig. 10) [35,49, 62,63]. Bone marrow involvement is an important indicator of the stage and prognosis in lymphoma, but diagnosis may be difficult to achieve by imaging or even by bone marrow biopsy, the latter of which is prone to sampling error within areas of inhomogeneous disease involvement [1]. The role

of FDG-PET in the evaluation of bone marrow involvement of lymphoma is controversial [8,12, 64,65]. The intramedullary localization of FDG uptake by PET/CT may be of potential value for guiding further diagnostic investigations, such as MRI or biopsy if indicated [33]. Stimulation of the bone marrow after the administration of granulocyte colony-stimulating factor can cause intense diffuse bone marrow uptake [49,66]. This transient uptake should not be mistaken for lymphoma involvement and usually resolves within up to 4 weeks after cessation of therapy [67].

Summary

In spite of the high performance of FDG-PET for the evaluation of lymphoma, inherent limitations of this modality underscore the additional value of PET/CT as an important tool in the assessment of this disease. Accumulating data on the use of PET/CT in lymphoma indicate the contribution of hybrid imaging to improved interpretation accuracy of PET using FDG and CT. Knowledge of the normal and abnormal patterns of FDG-PET/CT imaging and their variability in patients with lymphoma is important to provide a comprehensive clinically significant interpretation that has an impact on patient management and potentially on outcome.

References

[1] Vinnicombe SJ, Reznek RH. Computerised tomography in the staging of Hodgkin's disease and non-Hodgkin's lymphoma. Eur J Nucl Med Mol Imaging 2003;30(Suppl):S42–55.

[2] Kasamon YL, Wahl RL, Swinnen LJ. FDG PET and high-dose therapy for aggressive lymphomas: toward a risk-adapted strategy. Curr Opin Oncol 2004;16:100–5.

[3] Kostakoglu L, Goldsmith SJ. Fluorine-18 fluorodeoxyglucose positron emission tomography in the staging and follow-up of lymphoma: is it time to shift gears? Eur J Nucl Med 2000;27:1564–78.

[4] Sasaki M, Kuwabara Y, Koga H, et al. Clinical impact of whole body FDG-PET on the staging and therapeutic decision making for malignant lymphoma. Ann Nucl Med 2002;16:337–45.

[5] O'Doherty MJ, Macdonald EA, Barrington SF, et al. Positron emission tomography in the management of lymphomas. Clin Oncol 2002;14:415–26.

[6] Bar-Shalom R, Yefremov N, Haim N, et al. Camera-based FDG PET and 67Ga SPECT in evaluation of lymphoma: comparative study. Radiology 2003;227:353–60.

[7] Juweid ME, Cheson BD. Role of positron emission tomography in lymphoma. J Clin Oncol 2005;23:4577–80.

[8] Buchmann I, Reinhardt M, Elsner K, et al. 2-(fluorine-18)fluoro-2-deoxy-D-glucose positron emission tomography in the detection and staging of malignant lymphoma. A bicenter trial. Cancer 2001;91:889–99.

[9] Najjar F, Hustinx R, Jerusalem G, et al. Positron emission tomography (PET) for staging low-grade non-Hodgkin's lymphomas (NHL). Cancer Biother Radiopharm 2001;16:297–304.

[10] Schiepers C, Filmont JE, Czernin J. PET for staging of Hodgkin's disease and non-Hodgkin's lymphoma. Eur J Nucl Med Mol Imaging 2003;30(Suppl 1):S82–8.

[11] Blum RH, Seymour JF, Wirth A, et al. Frequent impact of F18-fluorodeoxyglucose positron emission tomography on the staging and management of patients with indolent non-Hodgkin's lymphoma. Clin Lymphoma 2003;4:43–9.

[12] Klose T, Leidl R, Buchmann I, et al. Primary staging of lymphomas: cost-effectiveness of FDG PET versus computed tomography. Eur J Nucl Med 2000;27:1457–64.

[13] Hicks RJ, Mac Manus MP, Seymour JF. Initial staging of lymphoma with positron emission tomography and computed tomography. Semin Nucl Med 2005;35:165–75.

[14] Spaepen K, Stroobants S, Dupont P, et al. Early restaging positron emission tomography with (18)F-fluorodeoxyglucose predicts outcome in patients with aggressive non-Hodgkin's lymphoma. Ann Oncol 2002;13:1356–63.

[15] Reinhardt MJ, Herkel C, Altehoefer C, et al. Computed tomography and 18F-FDG positron emission tomography for therapy control of Hodgkin's and non-Hodgkin's lymphoma patients: when do we really need FDG-PET? Ann Oncol 2005;16:1524–9.

[16] Juweid ME, Wiseman GA, Vose JM, et al. Response assessment of aggressive non-Hodgkin's lymphoma by integrated International Workshop Criteria and fluorine-18-fluorodeoxyglucose positron emission tomography. J Clin Oncol 2005;23:4652–61.

[17] Haioun C, Itti E, Rahmouni A, et al. [18F]fluoro-2-deoxy-D-glucose positron emission tomography (FDG-PET) in aggressive lymphoma: an early prognostic tool for predicting patient outcome. Blood 2005;106:1376–81.

[18] Schot B, van Imhoff G, Pruim J, et al. Predictive value of early 18F-fluoro-deoxyglucose positron emission tomography in chemosensitive relapsed lymphoma. Br J Haematol 2003;123:282–7.

[19] Jerusalem G, Hustinx R, Beguin Y, et al. Evaluation of therapy for lymphoma. Semin Nucl Med 2005;35:186–96.

[20] de Wit M, Bohuslavizki KH, Buchert R, et al. 18FDG-PET following treatment as valid predictor for disease-free survival in Hodgkin's lymphoma. Ann Oncol 2001;12:29–37.

[21] Jerusalem G, Beguin Y, Fassotte MF, et al. Early detection of relapse by whole-body positron emission tomography in the follow-up of patients with Hodgkin's disease. Ann Oncol 2003;14:123–30.

[22] Rigacci L, Castagnoli A, Dini C, et al. 18FDG-positron emission tomography in post treatment evaluation of residual mass in Hodgkin's lymphoma: long-term results. Oncol Rep 2005;14:1209–14.

[23] Castellucci P, Zinzani P, Pourdehnad M, et al. 18F-FDG PET in malignant lymphoma: significance of positive findings. Eur J Nucl Med Mol Imaging 2005;32:749–56.

[24] Surbone A, Longo DL, DeVita VT, et al. Residual abdominal masses in aggressive non-Hodgkin's lymphoma after combination chemotherapy: significance and management. J Clin Oncol 1988;6:1832–7.

[25] Jerusalem G, Beguin Y, Najjar F, et al. Positron emission tomography (PET) with F18-

fluorodeoxyglucose (F18-FDG) for the staging of low-grade non-Hodgkin's lymphoma (NHL). Ann Oncol 2001;12:825–30.

[26] Barrington SF, O'Doherty MJ. Limitations of PET for imaging lymphoma. Eur J Nucl Med Mol Imaging 2003;30(Suppl 1):S117–27.

[27] Kaste SC, Howard SC, McCarville EB, et al. 18F-FDG-avid sites mimicking active disease in pediatric Hodgkin's. Pediatr Radiol 2005;35: 141–54.

[28] Bar-Shalom R, Yefremov N, Guralnik L, et al. Clinical performance of PET/CT in evaluation of cancer: additional value for diagnostic imaging and patient management. J Nucl Med 2003;44:1200–9.

[29] Freudenberg LS, Antoch G, Schutt P, et al. FDG-PET/CT in re-staging of patients with lymphoma. Eur J Nucl Med Mol Imaging 2004;31:325–9.

[30] Schaefer NG, Hany TF, Taverna C, et al. Non-Hodgkin lymphoma and Hodgkin disease: coregistered FDG PET and CT at staging and restaging–do we need contrast-enhanced CT? Radiology 2004;232:823–9.

[31] Allen-Auerbach M, Quon A, Weber WA, et al. Comparison between 2-deoxy-2-[18F]fluoro-D-glucose positron emission tomography and positron emission tomography/computed tomography hardware fusion for staging of patients with lymphoma. Mol Imaging Biol 2004;6:411–6.

[32] Tatsumi M, Cohade C, Nakamoto Y, et al. Direct comparison of FDG PET and CT findings in patients with lymphoma: initial experience. Radiology 2005;237:1038–45.

[33] Rahmouni A, Luciani A, Itti E. MRI and PET in monitoring response in lymphoma. Cancer Imaging 2005;23(5 Suppl):S106–12.

[34] Schroder H, Larson SM, Yeung HW. PET/CT in oncology: integration into clinical management of lymphoma, melanoma, and gastrointestinal malignancies. J Nucl Med 2004;45(Suppl 1): 72S–81S.

[35] Blake MA, Slattery J, Sahani DV, et al. Practical issue in abdominal PET/CT. Appl Radiol 2005; 34:8–18.

[36] Moog F, Bangerter M, Diederichs CG, et al. Lymphoma: role of whole-body 2-deoxy-2-[F-18]fluoro-D-glucose (FDG) PET in nodal staging. Radiology 1997;203:795–800.

[37] Moog F, Bangerter M, Diederichs CG, et al. Extranodal malignant lymphoma: detection with FDG PET versus CT. Radiology 1998;206: 475–81.

[38] Young CS, Young BL, Smith SM. Staging Hodgkin's disease with FDG PET: comparison with CT and surgery. Clin Positron Imaging 1998;1: 161–4.

[39] Hueltenschmidt B, Sautter-Bihl ML, Lang O, et al. Whole body positron emission tomography in the management of Hodgkin's disease. Cancer 2001;91:302–10.

[40] Schroder H, Meta J, Yap C, et al. Effect of whole-body F18-FDG PET imaging on clinical staging and management of patients with malignant lymphoma. J Nucl Med 2001;42:1139–43.

[41] Wirth A, Seymour JF, Hicks RJ, et al. Fluorine-18 fluorodeoxyglucose positron emission tomography, gallium-67 scintigraphy, and conventional staging for Hodgkin's disease and non-Hodgkin's lymphoma. Am J Med 2002;112:262–8.

[42] de Juan R, Seifert B, Berthold T, et al. Clinical evaluation of a breathing protocol for PET/CT. Eur Radiol 2004;14:1118–23.

[43] Nehmeh SA, Erdi YE, Pan T, et al. Four-dimensional (4D) PET/CT imaging of the thorax. Med Phys 2004;31:3179–86.

[44] Elstrom R, Guan L, Baker G, et al. Utility of FDG-PET scanning in lymphoma by WHO classification. Blood 2003;101:3875–6.

[45] Jerusalem G, Beguin Y, Fassotte MF, et al. Whole-body positron emission tomography using 18F-fluorodeoxyglucose compared to standard procedures for staging patients with Hodgkin's disease. Haematologica 2001;86:266–73.

[46] Mikhaeel NG, Hutchings M, Fields PA, et al. FDG-PET after two to three cycles of chemotherapy predicts progression-free and overall survival in high-grade non-Hodgkin lymphoma. Ann Oncol 2005;16:1514–23.

[47] Brianzoni E, Rossi G, Ancidei S, et al. Radiotherapy planning: PET/CT scanner performances in the definition of gross tumour volume and clinical target volume. Eur J Nucl Med Mol Imaging 2005;32:1392–9.

[48] Schoder H, Noy A, Gonen M, et al. Intensity of 18-fluorodeoxyglucose uptake in positron emission tomography distinguishes between indolent and aggressive non-Hodgkin's lymphoma. J Clin Oncol 2005;23:4643–51.

[49] Cook GJ, Fogelman I, Maisey MN. Normal physiological and benign pathological variants of 18-fluoro-2-deoxyglucose positron-emission tomography scanning: potential for error in interpretation. Semin Nucl Med 1996;26: 308–14.

[50] Brink I, Reinhardt MJ, Hoegerle S, et al. Increased metabolic activity in the thymus gland studied with 18F-FDG PET: age dependency and frequency after chemotherapy. J Nucl Med 2001;42:591–5.

[51] Cohade C, Osman M, Pannu HK, et al. Uptake in supraclavicular area fat ("USA-Fat"): description on 18F-FDG PET/CT. J Nucl Med 2003;44: 170–6.

[52] Bar-Shalom R, Gaitini D, Keidar Z, et al. Non-malignant FDG uptake in infradiaphragmatic adipose tissue: a new site of physiological tracer biodistribution characterised by PET/CT. Eur J Nucl Med Mol Imaging 2004;31:1105–13.

[53] Jadvar H, Bonyadlou S, Iagaru A, et al. FDG PET-CT demonstration of Sjogren's sialoadenitis. Clin Nucl Med 2005;30:698–9.

[54] Bagheri B, Maurer AH, Cone L, et al. Characterization of the normal adrenal gland with 18F-FDG PET/CT. J Nucl Med 2004;45:1340–3.

[55] Kuo PH, Cooper DL, Cheng DW. Recurrence of lymphoma presenting as asymmetrically increased testicular activity on FDG-PET/CT. Semin Nucl Med 2006;36:105–7.

[56] Muylle K, Everaert H, De Mey J, et al. FDG accumulation in inguinal herniation mimicking metastatic disease. Clin Nucl Med 2004;29: 652–3.

[57] Lerman H, Metser U, Grisaru D, et al. Normal and abnormal F18-FDG endometrial and ovarian uptake in pre- and postmenopausal patients: assessment by PET/CT. J Nucl Med 2004;45: 266–71.

[58] Israel O, Yefremov N, Bar-Shalom R, et al. PET/CT detection of unexpected gastrointestinal foci of 18F-FDG uptake: incidence, localization patterns, and clinical significance. J Nucl Med 2005;46:758–62.

[59] Antoch G, Freudenberg LS, Stattaus J, et al. Whole-body positron emission tomography-CT: optimized CT using oral and IV contrast materials. AJR Am J Roentgenol 2002;179: 1555–60.

[60] Daldrup-Link HE, Franzius C, Link TM, et al. Whole-body MR imaging for detection of bone metastases in children and young adults:comparison with skeletal scintigraphy and FDG PET. AJR Am J Roentgenol 2001;177:229–36.

[61] Kanter P, Zeidman A, Streifler J, et al. PET-CT imaging of combined brachial and lumbosacral neurolymphomatosis. Eur J Haematol 2005;74: 66–9.

[62] Jacobsson H, Celsing F, Ingvar M, et al. Accumulation of FDG in axillary sweat glands in hyperhidrosis: a pitfall in whole-body PET examination. Eur Radiol 1998;8:482–3.

[63] Goerres GW, Ziegler SI, Burger C, et al. Artifacts at PET and PET/CT caused by metallic hip prosthetic material. Radiology 2003;226:577–84.

[64] Moog F, Bangerter M, Kotzerke J, et al. 18-F-fluorodeoxyglucose-positron emission tomography as a new approach to detect lymphomatous bone marrow. J Clin Oncol 1998;16:603–9.

[65] Pakos EE, Fotopoulos AD, Ioannidis JP. 18F-FDG PET for evaluation of bone marrow infiltration in staging of lymphoma: a meta-analysis. J Nucl Med 2005;46:958–63.

[66] Sugawara Y, Zasadny KR, Kison PV, et al. Splenic fluorodeoxyglucose uptake increased by granulocyte colony-stimulating factor therapy: PET imaging results. J Nucl Med 1999;40:1456–62.

[67] Sugawara Y, Fisher SJ, Zasadny KR, et al. Preclinical and clinical studies of bone marrow uptake of fluorine-1-fluorodeoxyglucose with or without granulocyte colony-stimulating factor during chemotherapy. J Clin Oncol 1998;16:173–80.

ELSEVIER
SAUNDERS

RADIOLOGIC
CLINICS
OF NORTH AMERICA

Radiol Clin N Am 45 (2007) 689–696

PET and PET/CT in Management of the Lymphomas

Donald A. Podoloff, MD[a],*, Homer A. Macapinlac, MD[b]

- F-18 fluorodeoxyglucose PET/CT at initial staging of lymphoma
- Response to treatment and prognosis evaluated with PET and PET/CT
- Incremental role of PET/CT in assessment of lymphoma
- PET and PET/CT in radiation therapy
- Summary
- References

It is estimated that there were approximately 7350 new cases and 1410 deaths from Hodgkin's disease (HD) in 2005 and approximately 56,000 new cases of non-Hodgkin's lymphoma (NHL) resulting in 19,200 deaths [1]. The incidence and death rate are equally distributed among men and women [1]. The incidence of NHL has increased steadily from 1975 to 2000, especially in people older than the age of 60 years, and approximately 140 new cases per 100,000 population older than the age of 60 years are now estimated [2]. With respect to prognostic factor modeling, patients can be separated into low-, intermediate-, and high-risk categories. The International Prognostic Index (IPI) is a useful tool for stratifying patients [3].

Compilation of multiple studies with as many as 1200 patients reported has demonstrated that there has been no change in the length of survival with NHL of the low-grade type over the years from 1960 to 1996, and no survival benefit was achieved by decade. Data from the M.D. Anderson Cancer Center on more than 400 patients demonstrate improved results in stage IV indolent lymphoma. In the time interval from 1977 to 1982, the medium length of survival was 7 years. From 1982 to

1988, the medium length of survival had increased to 11 years, and trends from 1988 through 1997 showed continuing improvement in survivorship, with the 50% survival not yet reached. These survival statistics, which are significantly different from those of other institutions, can largely be attributed to the fact that watchful waiting is rarely practiced in our patient population.

Lymphoma is a spectrum of malignant neoplasms of the lymphoid system. Their radiologic appearance is diverse, with almost all organs susceptible to involvement. The condition is challenging because it can mimic patterns of almost all other neoplasms [4]. If one considers the major modalities for imaging lymphoma, they can be divided into two general types. Radiography, CT, and MRI deal mostly with alterations of normal anatomy, detection of abnormal masses, and nodal enlargement. PET deals with alterations in biochemical processes and increased metabolism, such as glycolysis, amino acid transport, and DNA synthesis, depending on the tracer used.

PET and PET/CT with F-18 fluorodeoxyglucose (FDG) have been used as imaging modalities of lymphoma for the initial diagnosis and staging,

This article was previously published in PET Clinics 2006;1:243–50.
[a] Division of Diagnostic Imaging, University of Texas M.D. Anderson Cancer Center, 1515 Holcombe Boulevard, Houston, TX 77030, USA
[b] University of Texas M.D. Anderson Cancer Center, 1515 Holcombe Boulevard, Houston, TX 77030, USA
* Corresponding author.
E-mail address: dpodoloff@di.mdacc.tmc.edu (D.A. Podoloff).

doi:10.1016/j.rcl.2007.05.008

for therapeutic surveillance, to differentiate residual masses from fibrosis, and for prognostic purposes. These clinical applications are the major focus of this article.

F-18 fluorodeoxyglucose PET/CT at initial staging of lymphoma

At the University of Texas M.D. Anderson Cancer Center, clinical staging of HD and NHL begins with a detailed history and physical examination. Laboratory studies, including lactate dehydrogenase (LDH) and β-2 globulin, are important, especially for prognostic information. Routine chest radiography and CT with oral and intravenous contrast are performed from the neck to the pelvis. Bone marrow biopsy (BMB), PET, and, more recently, PET/CT are all part of the initial diagnostic workup of patients with lymphoma.

There may be significant improvements in patient outcome after the use of FDG-PET and PET/CT in lymphoma. One is the ability to upstage disease, and thus change the type and duration of therapy. Occasionally, patients are downstaged. The accuracy of metabolic staging of lymphoma has improved further after the introduction of PET/CT, because it has become possible to identify normal-sized hypermetabolic lymph nodes or lesions showing only slightly increased FDG uptake (Fig. 1).

As we move from an era of tissue identification to one of tissue characterization using radiopharmaceutic agents such as FDG, the ability to image on a more metabolic and molecular level is possible. How important this is in the lymphomas is

manifested by the fact that at our institution, where we perform more than 40 PET/CT scans a day, a little more than half are performed in patients from the lymphoma service, and this has held true over the past 5 years.

Several authors have extensively studied the performance of PET and PET/CT compared with CT over the past 5 years. Najjar and colleagues studied 36 patients with histologically proven low-grade NHL, including 21 patients in whom FDG-PET was performed at the time of initial diagnosis and 15 patients for restaging of disease recurrence, before any treatment. PET results were compared with those of physical examination and CT. An individual biopsy was available for a total of 31 lesions. The sensitivity and specificity were 87% and 100% for FDG-PET, 100% and 100% for physical examination, and 90% and 100% for CT, respectively. In addition, 42 of 97 peripheral lymph node lesions observed by FDG-PET were clinically undetected, whereas physical examination detected 23 additional nodal lesions. PET and CT indicated 12 extranodal lymphomatous localizations. FDG-PET showed 7 additional extranodal lesions, whereas 5 additional unconfirmed lesions were observed on CT. Regarding bone marrow infiltration, PET and biopsy were concordant in 24 patients, with 11 true-positive (TP) and 13 true-negative (TN) studies. PET resulted in false-negative (FN) studies in 11 patients, however [5].

The combined assessment, including PET/CT and physical examination, seems to be more sensitive than the conventional approach for staging low-grade NHL. Its sensitivity, however, is unacceptably low for diagnosing bone marrow infiltration.

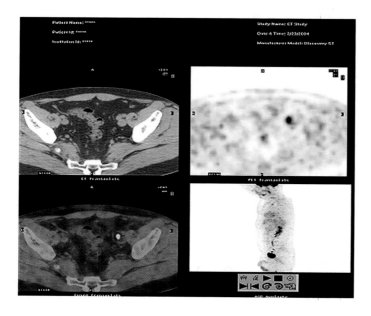

Fig. 1. Hypermetabolic normal-sized left iliac node in a 62-year-old patient with large B-cell NHL.

Buchmann and coworkers [6] undertook a prospective evaluation of the clinical value of FDG-PET in the detection and staging of malignant lymphoma compared with CT and BMB. They studied 52 consecutive patients with untreated malignant lymphoma, investigating lymph node and/or extranodal manifestations and bone marrow infiltration. Discrepant results were verified by biopsy, MRI, or clinical follow-up. A total of 1297 anatomic regions (lymph nodes, organs, and bone marrow) were evaluated. FDG-PET and CT scans were compared by receiver operating characteristic (ROC) curve analysis. The area under the ROC curve was as follows: for lymph nodes, 0.996 (PET) and 0.916 (CT); for extranodal lymphoma, 0.999 (PET) and 0.916 (CT); for supradiaphragmatic involvement, 0.996 (PET) and 0.905 (CT); and for infradiaphragmatic disease, 0.999 (PET) and 0.952 (CT). FDG-PET was significantly superior to CT ($P<.05$), except for the infradiaphragmatic regions, in which the two methods produced equivalent results. In detecting bone marrow infiltration, FDG-PET was superior to CT and equivalent to BMB. In 8% of patients, FDG-PET led to upstaging of disease and subsequent change in therapy. FDG-PET thus seems to be an accurate noninvasive modality for the staging of lymphoma, which is significantly superior when compared with standard staging modalities, including CT and BMB. In a prospective study, Bangerter and colleagues [7] evaluated 44 patients with newly diagnosed HD and NHL. They compared conventional imaging (CT and ultrasound) with PET. PET determined a change of stage in 14% of cases, mainly by upstaging disease. A similar study by Young and coworkers [8] in 45 newly diagnosed and 4 relapsed HD cases demonstrated that PET upstaged 21 patients, equally staged 16 patients, and downstaged 1 patient as compared with CT.

Foo and colleagues [9] reported a retrospective study of 38 patients who had FDG-PET scans: 24 at initial staging and 46 at restaging. Performance of PET was compared with concurrent gallium-67 scans and CT, with disease validation by clinical follow-up or biopsy. The sensitivities of PET and CT at initial staging were 96% and 71%, respectively. PET identified additional sites of disease compared with CT in 29% of patients. In patients who had all three imaging modalities, the sensitivities of PET, CT, and gallium scintigraphy were 93%, 67%, and 87%, respectively.

Response to treatment and prognosis evaluated with PET and PET/CT

FDG-PET and PET/CT are diagnostic procedures that have assumed an important role in the management of patients with lymphoma because of the prognostic information that they can provide, and because, at present, there are multiple therapeutic alternatives available in management of the different histologic types of lymphoma (Fig. 2). As a rule, patients with NHL are reimaged after short intervals (as often as every 6 weeks) with PET/CT, including the neck, chest, abdomen, and pelvis.

PET and PET/CT are better discriminators than CT with respect to disease-free interval and overall survival. It is important to recognize that although PET and PET/CT are valuable adjuncts in restaging and prognosis, meticulous attention to detail and consistency of technique is important to interpret these studies properly.

With respect to prognosis, Spaepen and coworkers [10] demonstrated the survival advantage in a group of 93 patients defined by PET imaging performed at 1 to 3 months after first-line chemotherapy. PET-negative patients had a much longer progression-free survival as compared with PET-positive patients. A prospective study showed that the addition of PET results to clinical criteria provided a more accurate treatment response classification in patients with aggressive NHL as compared with the use of clinical prognostic indices alone [11].

The predictive role of PET in determining the outcome of lymphoma patients was assessed as well. After treatment, 4 (80%) of 5 patients who were PET-positive and CT-negative relapsed as compared with none of 29 patients in the PET- and CT-negative subset. Among the 41 CT-positive patients, 91% who were also PET-positive relapsed as compared with none of the PET-negative patients. The relapse-free survival rates were 9% and 100% in the PET-positive and PET-negative subsets, respectively ($P = .00001$). Five patients who were PET-positive and CT-negative underwent lymph node biopsy; in 4 of these patients, persistent viable lymphoma was confirmed at histopathologic examination. Conversely, 2 patients who were PET-negative and CT-positive, with large residual masses in the mediastinum or lungs, also underwent biopsy, which revealed only fibrosis in both cases. The authors concluded that in HD and aggressive NHL patients, PET positivity after induction treatment is highly predictive for the presence of residual disease, with significant differences in relapse-free survival. PET negativity at restaging strongly suggests the absence of active disease [12].

The diagnostic accuracy of FDG-PET in detecting residual viable disease or relapse during the post-therapy period was assessed in 48 patients with HD and compared with CT. Different predictive values for FDG-PET were found according to the time interval between the end of therapy and the PET study [13]. Results of PET and CT were compared with clinical follow-up, with relapse being

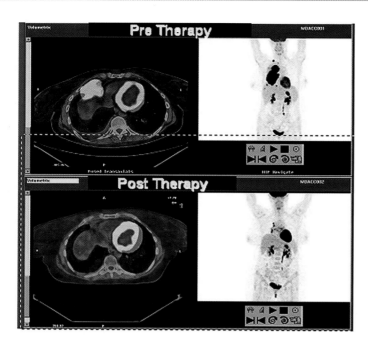

Fig. 2. Metabolic response after only two cycles of rituximab plus CHOP in a 41-year-old patient with mediastinal diffuse large B-cell NHL.

defined by a positive biopsy or the introduction of a second-line treatment. The sensitivity and specificity of FDG-PET to predict relapse were 79% and 97%, respectively. The positive predictive value (PPV) and negative predictive value (NPV) were both equal to 92%. The diagnostic accuracy of FDG-PET (92%) was significantly higher than the accuracy of CT (56%) ($P < .005$). Patients with positive FDG-PET studies had a far shorter median disease-free interval (79 days) than those with positive CT studies (disease-free proportion of 52% at 1143 days) ($P = .0046$). Three false-negative FDG-PET studies were found in patients who underwent their PET study within the first 49 days after the end of chemotherapy [13].

A large cohort of patients whose management after induction therapy was based on routine PET and CT restaging was reported on by Zinzani and colleagues [14]. Fifty-nine patients with HD or aggressive NHL presenting with abdominal involvement (35% with bulky disease) were studied with PET and CT after combined chemotherapy and radiation treatment. After treatment, all 3 patients who were PET-positive/CT-negative relapsed as compared with none of 7 patients in the PET-negative/CT-negative subset. Among the 49 patients who were CT-positive, 60% who were PET-positive relapsed as compared with 5% who were PET-negative. The relapse-free survival rates were 0% in the PET-positive/CT-negative subset and 100% in the PET-negative/CT-negative subset, respectively. PET restaging seems to be valuable for the identification

of patients who would need appropriate second-line therapy because of the presence of residual active abdominal disease and should be made widely available in combination with CT. The role of PET in defining the nature of residual mass identified on CT at the end of treatment was evaluated in 58 patients with HD and NHL who had achieved complete remission after therapy. The PET-positive recurrence rate was 62.5% as compared with an incidence of PET-negative recurrence less than 4% [15].

Dittmann and coworkers [16] performed a blind comparative analysis of the results of CT and FDG-PET with respect to the viability of residual masses and in cases of suspected relapse. PET was assessed visually and by quantifying FDG activity using the standard uptake value (SUV). Changes in the size of tumor lesions as well as contrast medium enhancement served as criteria for assessment by CT. FDG-PET showed an increased tracer uptake in studies of 8 of 26 residual lesions, of which 7 were TP and 1 was false positive (FP). Eighteen cases showed no FDG uptake and were classified as showing no viable HD, with 17 TN and 1 FN studies. In the blinded reading of the corresponding CT studies, 10 cases were further shown to contain viable lymphoma (2 TP and 8 FP studies). Sixteen CT studies were classified as negative (10 TP and 6 FN studies). The sensitivity and specificity of PET were 87.5% and 94.4% in contrast to only 25% and 56% for CT. The PPV and NPV of PET and CT were 87.5% and 94.4% as compared with 20%

and 62.5%, respectively. In patients with suspected relapse, the sensitivity and PPV for the diagnosis of recurrence were 100% and 86%, respectively, equal for both methods. In HD with residual masses after treatment, FDG-PET seems to offer important additional information regarding the presence of viable disease in these lesions. In patients with suspected relapse of HD, FDG-PET seems not to offer any information over CT scans. Quantitative assessment using SUVs was not found to be superior to visual assessment of PET.

A study published in the *Annals of Oncology* in 2002 addressed the issue of early restaging in NHL [17]. In a study with 70 patients treated with doxorubicin (cyclophosphamide, doxorubicin, vincristine, and prednisone [CHOP]/variance), none of 33 patients with persistent positive PET studies at midtreatment had durable complete remission, whereas 31 of 37 patients with negative PET studies had no evidence of disease for a follow-up with a medium duration of 1107 days, with the 6 additional patients showing only a partial response or relapse. These authors thus concluded that midtreatment PET results represented a stronger prognostic factor for disease-free and overall survival than the clinical pretreatment factors included in the IPI [17].

Hart and colleagues [18] addressed the issue of the utility of FDG-PET in lymphoma patients who had undergone allografting for their disease. PET was of value in determining when donor lymphocytes should be infused after therapy. This retrospective pilot study forms the basis of a prospective study to clarify the utility of PET imaging in these patients.

The role of imaging in the assessment of response to treatment in patients with central nervous system lymphoma is somewhat controversial. High FDG metabolism can be seen in high-grade gliomas and in infectious diseases (Fig. 3). It is appreciated, however, that metabolic PET imaging and PET/CT can guide stereotactic biopsies to be used for further assessment of treatment response [19].

Incremental role of PET/CT in assessment of lymphoma

The addition of CT to PET has several advantages. It provides for anatomic localization of hypermetabolic areas, and it allows for more rapid imaging, because the attenuation correction can be accomplished quicker, especially with multidetector CT scanners.

There are significant pitfalls with respect to FDG imaging, which are more evident and of higher clinical significance after treatment. Small lesions less than 6 mm may not be resolved, especially at the

lung basis. Lesions with a diameter of approximately 10 mm may not be seen in the brain and in the liver because of high glucose uptake in surrounding tissues. The differential diagnosis between bone marrow hyperplasia attributable to associated treatment with colony-stimulating factor and diffuse bone marrow involvement is sometimes difficult.

Peritoneal lesions may be missed because of their small size or if there is diffuse uptake, but they are often visible on the CT portion of a PET/CT study, even when contrast material is not used. Additional pitfalls may occur, because many FDG-avid lesions can be benign; among them are infectious processes, tuberculosis, and sarcoid lesion. There are also occasional lesions that do not take up large amounts of FDG, such as mantle cell and marginal zone lymphoma (as well as Richter's transformation in our experience).

An additional piece of information that is provided by PET and PET/CT scanning is insight into the heterogeneous nature of some of the tumors. Masses that appear relatively homogeneous on non–contrast-enhanced CT may be quite variable with respect to their glucose uptake (Fig. 4).

The availability of anatomic mapping provides topographic landmarks that may be used for functional guiding of biopsy, which may allow for the differential diagnosis between lymphoma tissue and one of the previously mentioned benign conditions associated with FDG avidity. PET/CT may also allow pinpointing further invasive assessment to hypermetabolic lesions, and thus differentiating between residual masses and residual viable tumor.

Confusion in the clinic can also be caused by radiation effects, especially early after therapy. An article by Castellucci and coworkers [20] reported on 16 consecutive patients assessed early, however, at 1 to 2 months after radiation therapy using PET. Only 3 of the 16 patients had mild uptake in areas of previous radiation, and none of these findings would have been confused with disease. Even in problematic cases, however, the availability of anatomic images that may allow for identification of characteristic radiation-induced patterns of changes in structural features may help to resolve this diagnostic dilemma.

PET, CT, and PET/CT hardware fusion were compared in 73 patients with HD or NHL who underwent staging with an integrated PET/CT system. A discordant image interpretation between PET and PET/CT occurred in 10% of patients. PET/CT correctly upstaged 2 patients and downstaged 5 patients. Overall staging was accurate in 93% of patients with PET/CT and in 84% with PET (*P* = .03), with these results thus demonstrating a higher lymphoma staging accuracy using PET/CT as compared with PET alone [21].

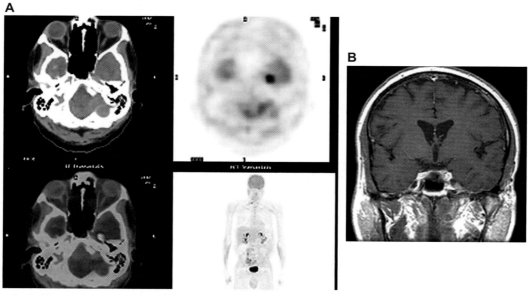

Fig. 3. A 45-year-old man with a history of gastric lymphoma treated with CHOP chemotherapy developed numbness, diplopia, and tongue deviation. A cerebrospinal fluid sample demonstrated the presence of lymphoma cells. The results of brain MRI were reported as normal. (*A*) FDG-PET/CT study demonstrates a hypermetabolic focus in the left hemisphere. The presence of a subtle but active focus on PET induced repeat evaluation of the MRI study. (*B*) T1-weighted coronal MRI slice demonstrates subtle abnormal enhancement in the inferior aspect of Meckel's cave on the left side, consistent with subarachnoid lymphoma.

The improved ability to localize anatomic detail by the combination of PET/CT has provided much useful information in the assessment of cancer patients. Nevertheless, there is controversy as to the absolute necessity of combining PET and CT in patients with lymphoma. The group at the University Hospital in Zurich published an article suggesting that the CT added little when combined with PET in the assessment of lymphoma [22], whereas, more recently, the group at The Johns Hopkins University presented contrary evidence suggesting that

there was significant incremental value provided by PET/CT in the assessment of lymphoma, because hybrid imaging added certainty and allowed for better diagnosis as compared with stand-alone PET [23].

An additional issue was recently assessed in a retrospective review that compared the diagnostic value of low-dose nonenhanced CT coregistered to FDG-PET (PET/CT) with the results of routinely obtained high-resolution contrast-enhanced CT for staging and restaging of disease in 60 patients

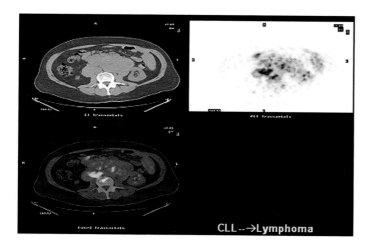

Fig. 4. Inhomogeneous FDG uptake in a viable lymphoma mass that appears homogeneous on the noncontrast CT scan in a 67-year-old patient with chronic lymphocytic lymphoma, which transformed to B-cell NHL.

with HD or high-grade NHL. For evaluation of lymph node involvement, the sensitivities of PET/CT and contrast-enhanced CT were 94% and 88% and the specificities were 100% and 86%, respectively. For the evaluation of organ involvement, the sensitivities of PET/CT and contrast-enhanced CT were 88% and 50% and the specificities were 100% and 90%, respectively. Agreement of both methods was excellent for assignment of lymph node involvement but was only fair for extranodal disease. PET/CT performed with nonenhanced CT was thus more sensitive and specific than contrast-enhanced CT for evaluation of lymph node and organ involvement in lymphoma as well as for exclusion of disease in suspicious sites [22].

The M.D. Anderson experience with more than 15,000 PET studies suggests that the combination of PET/CT is of particular value when involved lymph nodes are normal in size or when imaging in a complicated anatomic area (eg, head and neck, pelvis) and that it helps to increase the diagnostic certainty of the interpreter.

PET and PET/CT in radiation therapy

PET and especially PET/CT are useful for abdominal lymphoma patients and may be quite useful in the context of radiation therapy, where FDG-PET provides unique information on the presence of residual active disease. A recent review by Hutchings and coworkers [24] summarized the impact of combined PET/CT in radiation planning and concluded that few data have thus far been published allowing anything more than an expectation that because PET/CT provides anatomic and functional information in a fused format, it should be superior to PET or CT alone. To date, intuition rather than science would predict that such fusion would lead to decreased toxicity and improved therapeutic outcomes.

Summary

Within recent years, FDG-PET has become the most important nuclear medicine and radiology imaging modality in the management of lymphoma. FDG-PET detects more disease sites and involved organs than conventional staging procedures, including CT, and has a large influence on staging. FDG-PET performed during and after therapy seems to provide considerable prognostic information. The impact on patient outcome is not clear, however, because no controlled trials have yet been conducted and follow-up periods are generally short.

Nevertheless, the extraordinary rapid acceptance of this combined modality in the clinic and its total replacement of PET-only imaging in our institution as well as in others suggest that PET/CT may have even more impact on clinical management than did CT and MRI when they were introduced. Now that we understand the basic cause of cancer is genetic origin, we are beginning to understand that only by imaging such changes at the molecular level can we hope to influence the final outcome of this disease. Lymphomas represent an excellent model on which to focus, because we already know so much about the genetic alterations that lead to them.

References

[1] Jemal A, Murray T, Ward E, et al. Cancer statistics. CA Cancer J Clin 2005;55(1):10–30.

[2] Weir R, Thun MJ, Hankey BF et al. SEER cancer statistics review 1975–2000. Bethesda (MD): National Cancer Institute.

[3] Bastion Y, Berger F, Bryon PA, et al. Follicular lymphomas; assessment of prognostic factors in 127 patients followed for 10 years. Ann Oncol 1991;(Suppl 2):123–9.

[4] Haliday T, Baxter G. Lymphoma. Pictorial review II. Eur Radiol 2003;13:1224–34.

[5] Hustinx R, Jerusalem G, Fillet G, et al. Positron emission tomography (PET) for staging low-grade non-Hodgkin's lymphomas (NHL). Cancer Biother Radiopharm 2001;16:297–304.

[6] Buchmann I, Reinhardt M, Elsner K, et al. 2-(fluorine-18)fluoro-2-deoxy-D-glucose positron emission tomography in the detection and staging of malignant lymphoma. A bicenter trial. Cancer 2001;91:889–99.

[7] Bangerter M, Moog F, Buchman I, et al. Whole-body 2-[18F]-fluoro-2-deoxy-D-glucose positron emission tomography (FDG-PET) for accurate staging of Hodgkin's disease. Ann Oncol 1998; 9:1117–22.

[8] Young CS, Young BL, Smith SM. Staging Hodgkin's disease with 18-FDG PET. Clin Positron Imaging 1998;1:161–4.

[9] Foo SS, Mitchell PL, Berlangieri SU, et al. Positron emission tomography scanning in the assessment of patients with lymphoma. Int Med J 2004;34:388–97.

[10] Spaepen K, Stroobants S, Dupont P, et al. Prognostic value of positron emission tomography (PET) with fluorine-18 fluorodeoxyglucose (18F-FDG) after first-line chemotherapy in non-Hodgkin's lymphoma: is 18F-FDG-PEY a valid alternative to conventional diagnostic methods? J Clin Oncol 2001;192:414–9.

[11] Juweid ME, Wiseman GA, Vose JM, et al. Response assessment of aggressive non-Hodgkin's lymphoma by integrated International Workshop Criteria and fluorine-18-fluorodeoxyglucose positron emission tomography. J Clin Oncol 2005;23:4652–61.

[12] Zinzani PL, Fanti S, Battista G, et al. Predictive role of positron emission tomography (PET) in

the outcome of lymphoma patients. Br J Cancer 2004;91:850–4.

[13] Guay C, Lepine M, Verreault J, et al. Prognostic value of PET using 18F-FDG in Hodgkin's disease for post treatment evaluation. J Nucl Med 2003;44:1225–31.

[14] Zinzani PL, Chierichetti F, Zompatori M, et al. Advantages of positron emission tomography (PET) with respect to computed tomography in the follow-up of lymphoma patients with abdominal presentation. Leuk Lymphoma 2002;43:1239–43.

[15] Naumann R, Vaic A, Beuthien-Baumann B, et al. Prognostic value of positron emission tomography in the evaluation of post-treatment residual mass in patients with Hodgkin's disease and non-Hodgkin's lymphoma. Br J Hematol 2001; 115:793–800.

[16] Dittmann H, Sokler M, Kollmannsberger C, et al. Comparison of 18FDG-PET with CT scans in the evaluation of patients with residual and recurrent Hodgkin's lymphoma. Oncol Rep 2001;8: 1393–9.

[17] Spaepen K, Stroobants S, Dupont P, et al. Early restaging positron emission tomography with 18F-fluorodeoxuglucose predicts outcome in patients with aggressive non-Hodgkin's lymphoma. Ann Oncol 2002;13:1356–63.

[18] Hart DP, Avivi I, Thomson KJ, et al. Use of 18F-FDG positron emission tomography following allergenic transplantation to guide adoptive immunotherapy with donor lymphocyte infusions. Br J Haematol 2005;128:824–9.

[19] Roelke U, Leenders KL. Positron emission tomography in patients with primary CNS lymphomas. J Neurooncol 1999;43:231–6.

[20] Castellucci P, Zinzani P, Nanni C, et al. 18F-FDG PET early after radiotherapy in lymphoma patients. Cancer Biother Radiopharm 2004;19: 606–12.

[21] Allen-Auerbach M, Quon A, Weber WA, et al. Comparison between 2-deoxy-2-[18F]fluoro-D-glucose positron emission tomography and positron emission tomography/computed tomography hardware fusion for staging of patients with lymphoma. Mol Imaging Biol 2004;6:411–6.

[22] Schaefer NG, Hany TF, Taverna C, et al. Non-Hodgkin's lymphoma and Hodgkin's disease: co-registered FDG PET and CT at staging and restaging—do we need contrast-enhanced CT? Radiology 2004;232:823–9.

[23] Tatsumi M, Cohade C, Nakamoto Y, et al. Direct comparison of FDG PET and CT findings in patients with lymphoma: initial experience. Radiology 2005;237:1038–45.

[24] Hutchings M, Eigtved AI, Specht L. FDG-PET in the clinical management of Hodgkin lymphoma. Crit Rev Oncol Hemat 2004;52:19–32.

RADIOLOGIC
CLINICS
OF NORTH AMERICA

Radiol Clin N Am 45 (2007) 697–709

Fluorine-18 Fluorodeoxyglucose PET/CT Patterns of Extranodal Involvement in Patients with Non-Hodgkin Lymphoma and Hodgkin's Disease

Einat Even-Sapir, MD, PhD[a],*, Genady Lievshitz, MD[a],
Chava Perry, MD[b], Yair Herishanu, MD[b], Hedva Lerman, MD[a],
Ur Metser, MD[a]

- Fluorine-18 fluorodeoxyglucose PET and PET/CT in extranodal lymphoma: overview
- Fluorine-18 fluorodeoxyglucose PET/CT in marginal zone lymphomas
- Lymphoma of the gastrointestinal tract and abdominal and pelvic organs
- Lymphoma of the head and neck
- Lymphoma in the region of the thorax
- Lymphoma involving the bone marrow and cortical bone
- Lymphoma involving the nervous system
- Summary
- References

Non-Hodgkin lymphoma (NHL) may arise in nodal and extranodal sites. The term *non-lymph node nodal* lymphoma refers to certain lymphomas located in Waldeyer's ring, the thymus, and the spleen. Extranodal lymphoma (ENL) may arise along the gastrointestinal tract (GIT), head and neck, orbit, central nervous system (CNS) and peripheral nervous system, lung and pleura, bone, skin, breast, testis, thyroid, and genitourinary tract (GUT) [1]. When lymphoma involves extranodal sites, it is of importance to determine whether the tumor originated in nonnodal tissue (primary ENL), whether it originated in nodal tissue and spread to adjacent nonnodal tissue, or whether it

originated in nodal tissue and hematogenously spread to extranodal sites (secondary ENL) [2]. Accurate localization of disease is essential for appropriate treatment strategy, which may be related to organ-specific problems [1,3]. Moreover, extranodal involvement is among the well-established pretreatment prognostic factors in patients with lymphoma [4].

The incidence of NHL has increased over the past 2 decades and at a more significant pace for extranodal disease as compared with nodal disease [1,5]. Potential explanations for this epidemiologic phenomenon are the AIDS epidemic and other viral infections, an increase in the number of patients

This article was previously published in PET Clinics 2006;1:251–65.
[a] Department of Nuclear Medicine, Tel-Aviv Sourasky Medical Center, Sackler Faculty of Medicine, Tel-Aviv University, 6 Weizman Street, Tel-Aviv 64239, Israel
[b] Department of Hematology, Tel-Aviv Sourasky Medical Center, Sackler Faculty of Medicine, Tel-Aviv University, 6 Weizman Street, Tel-Aviv 64239, Israel
* Corresponding author.
E-mail address: evensap@tasmc.health.gov.il (E. Even-Sapir).

exposed to previous immunosuppressive treatment, and altered environmental conditions [1]. At least one quarter of NHLs arise primarily at extranodal sites. Summarizing the database on 91,306 patients with NHL, Glass and colleagues [2] reported extranodal NHL to form 28% of all cases and 15% in the case of low-grade histology. In another series on 318 patients with NHL, 46% had primary ENL. The stomach was the most common extranodal site, followed by the skin and head and neck region. Compared with nodal disease, primary ENLs tend to be localized and to have extranodal relapses more often [6]. Aggressive types of lymphoma, mainly diffuse large B-cell lymphoma (DLCL), predominate histologically in ENL, followed by follicular lymphomas. There are other subtypes of lymphoma, however, such as mucosa-associated lymphoid tissue (MALT) lymphomas and mantle cell lymphomas, which, overall, are less common lymphoma subtypes but are associated with a high incidence of extranodal involvement [7–9]. Being the third most frequent histologic subtype, MALT lymphoma, an ENL originating in marginal zone (MZ) cells, accounts for only 8% of all NHL cases but for almost half of primary gastric lymphomas [1]. The mantle cell subtype accounts for 5% to 10% of NHL cases, with an overall poor prognosis. Frequently, disease is disseminated, involving the lymph nodes, bone marrow, spleen, and extranodal sites. In a report on 121 patients with mantle cell lymphoma, 96 had bone marrow disease, 58 had splenic involvement, 21 had GIT disease, 15 had involvement of the liver, 14 had lymphoma in the head and neck, 9 had lymphoma in the pleura and/or lung, and 10 had involvement of other extranodal sites [10].

Hodgkin's disease (HD) is usually confined to the lymph nodes. Extranodal involvement is much less common in HD compared with NHL. Extranodal involvement is more often attributable to direct extension from adjacent nodal disease. Hematogenous spread has been reported during the course of the disease in 5% to 10% of the patients, however. According to the Ann Arbor classification of lymphoma, "E" defines the involvement of a single extralymphatic site or a contiguous extranodal extension in proximity to a known nodal site. Disseminated involvement of one or more organs or tissues, with or without associated lymph node involvement, is termed stage IV disease and is associated with a less favorable outcome [11].

Fluorine-18 fluorodeoxyglucose PET and PET/CT in extranodal lymphoma: overview

Before the fluorine-18 fluorodeoxyglucose (^18F-FDG) PET era, staging of lymphoma was based on physical examination and morphologic imaging, mainly using CT. CT has a limited sensitivity in detecting lymphomatous involvement of normal-sized lymph nodes, bone marrow, and spleen, however. CT may show nonspecific findings suggestive of extranodal sites of disease; therefore, it often requires further validation [3]. In a recent meta-analysis of 20 publications that assessed the role of ^18F-FDG PET in staging lymphoma, it was shown that PET upstaged disease in 8% to 17% of patients and downstaged disease in 2% to 23% of patients [12]. Several studies have specifically addressed the superiority of ^18F-FDG PET over CT for assessment of extranodal involvement [13–16]. Moog and co-workers [13] reported that in 16% of the patients (43 with NHL and 38 with HD), PET modified staging as compared with CT by detecting unsuspected involvement of the spleen, liver, and bone or by excluding disease in false-positive CT lesions. Rodriguez and colleagues [17] reported detection of greater extension by PET compared with endoscopy and CT in patients with high-grade lymphoma of the stomach. In another study by Schaefer and co-workers [18] on 60 patients with lymphoma, PET/CT was found to be more sensitive than full-dose contrast-enhanced CT in identification of nodal and extranodal sites of disease. For extranodal involvement, the sensitivity and specificity were 88% and 100%, respectively, for PET/CT and 50% and 90%, respectively, for contrast-enhanced CT. In a recent report by Raanani and colleagues [16], the diagnostic accuracy of PET/CT and diagnostic CT were compared in 103 consecutive patients with newly diagnosed NHL and HD. Upstaging disease by PET/CT was observed mostly in patients in stages I and II, detecting involvement in small-sized lymph nodes as well as in the spleen, liver, thymus, cortical bone, bone marrow, lung, and pleura, sites that were overlooked when CT was interpreted alone.

^18F-FDG avidity is a hallmark for the accurate staging of lymphoma using ^18F-FDG PET/CT. High-grade lymphomas are usually ^18F-FDG–avid, as are many cases of follicular type lymphomas. ^18F-FDG avidity of marginal zone lymphomas (MZLs), the third most common lymphoma type in extranodal lesions, is a controversial issue, however.

Fluorine-18 fluorodeoxyglucose PET/CT in marginal zone lymphomas

The secondary B follicle found in the lymph nodes, spleen, and ENL tissue is composed of a follicle center and the mantle, which comprises the lymphocytic corona and the MZ. The MZ is developed in the spleen, Payer's patches, and tonsils, which are secondary lymphoid organs, and is poorly developed in peripheral lymph nodes. There are three subtypes of lymphomas originating in the MZ:

nodal (monocytoid) MZ lymphoma, splenic MZ lymphoma, and extranodal MZ lymphoma (also referred as MALT lymphoma). Osaacson and Wright defined MALT lymphoma as a distinct entity in 1983 [7,8]. MALT lymphoma was originally identified in the GIT but was later identified in the lung and salivary and lacrimal duct mucosa as well and then in other sites normally devoid of MALT, where MALT is acquired in response to antigenic stimulation, such as Hashimoto's thyroiditis, Sjögren's syndrome, and gastric *Helicobacter pylori*. There is compelling evidence implicating *H pylori* in the pathogenesis of gastric lymphoma, which is the most common site of MALT lymphoma [1,7,8,19]. Nongastric MALT lymphoma may involve the skin, thyroid, breast, thymus, orbit, liver, kidney, prostate, urinary bladder, and gallbladder [7,8,19]. Disseminated disease is common in MALT lymphoma, where 25% of patients have involvement of multiple mucosal sites and/or involvement of nonmucosal sites, such as the bone marrow [20]. MALT lymphoma has generally been considered as non-^{18}F-FDG–avid. In a preliminary study, Hoffman and colleagues [21] assessed the role of PET for the staging of MALT lymphoma in 21 patients and reported a difference in ^{18}F-FDG avidity between nodal MZL, with PET-positive studies in 5 of 6 patients, as compared with negative studies in all patients with MALT lymphoma. The authors therefore suggested the potential use of ^{18}F-FDG PET for differentiating nodal and extranodal MZL. Opposite conclusions were suggested recently by Beal and coworkers [22], who reported on 175 patients with biopsy-proven MALT lymphoma. Of 42 patients who underwent PET for initial staging, 34 (81%) had ^{18}F-FDG–avid disease, 6 (14%) had non-^{18}F-FDG–avid disease, and 2 (5%) showed indeterminate uptake. Based on PET assessment, regional nodal involvement was found in 21% of the patients with ^{18}F-FDG–avid disease. In 4 patients, disease was upstaged based on unexpected PET findings. Follow-up PET was found to be accurate in differentiating complete response from active disease [22]. The authors thus concluded that ^{18}F-FDG PET is a valuable imaging modality for staging and for monitoring response to therapy of MALT lymphoma. Other reports, mainly case studies, have described ^{18}F-FDG–avid MALT lymphomas. MALT lymphoma of the lung, for example, was reported to present occasionally as a solitary ^{18}F-FDG–avid lesion, and the authors thus suggested the inclusion of this entity in the differential diagnosis of indeterminate lung lesions showing increased tracer uptake [23].

It is not clear why some cases of MALT lymphoma would show increased uptake of ^{18}F-FDG, whereas others would not. MZLs display a broad morphologically heterogeneous composite of cells that include small B cells (centrocyte-like cells, monocytoid cells, and small lymphocytes), large B cells, and plasma cells [8]. This heterogeneity of the cellular composition may be the potential cause for differences in ^{18}F-FDG avidity. It should be noted that in previous publications on MALT lymphoma, PET was usually the technology performed rather than PET/CT. It is therefore yet to be determined whether the use PET/CT may improve the diagnostic accuracy of ^{18}F-FDG PET in detecting MALT lymphomas, particularly in tissue in which uptake may be found physiologically, such as the GIT (Fig. 1).

Lymphoma of the gastrointestinal tract and abdominal and pelvic organs

The GIT is the most common extranodal site in NHL, accounting for approximately 10% to 15% of all NHLs and 30% to 40% of all extranodal cases [1]. Any region along the GIT, from the oral cavity to the anus, may be involved by lymphoma, with the stomach and small intestine being the most common sites. Lymphoma of the stomach comprises 1% to 10% of all gastric malignancies. It may be limited disease localized to the stomach and perigastric lymph nodes or advanced disease (Fig. 2) [1,23–25]. Small intestinal lymphoma represents 36% to 54% of all GIT lymphomas and 18% to 24% of all small bowel malignancies. Lymphoma types involving the small intestine are usually DLCL and MALT lymphoma [25–27]. Patients with celiac disease have an increased risk of developing enteropathy-associated T-cell lymphoma [1]. Involvement of the GIT by HD is uncommon. When the GIT is involved, it is usually by extension from adjacent lymph nodes [11].

Encouraging results have been reported by Kumar and colleagues [26] when PET was used to differentiate residual or recurrent disease and nonactive masses in patients with GIT lymphomas, with a positive predictive value (PPV) of 100% and a negative predictive value (NPV) of 92%. Physiologic uptake of ^{18}F-FDG along the GIT may lead to false-positive and false-negative interpretations of PET in patients with GIT lymphoma, however, particularly in the presence of minimal disease [13]. PET/CT may improve the differentiation between physiologic ^{18}F-FDG uptake from uptake in lymphoma, as was illustrated in a pictorial assay on PET/CT in ENL cases [28]. Oral administration of contrast media seems to be beneficial in patients with GIT lymphoma, allowing for better delineation of the stomach or bowel wall on the CT part of the PET/CT study (see Fig. 2; Fig. 3) [29].

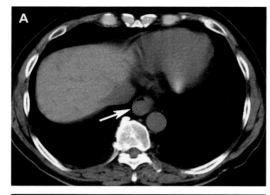

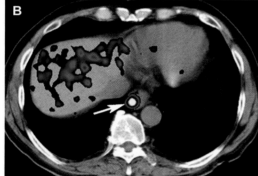

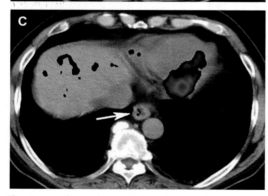

Fig. 1. Esophageal MALT lymphoma. At diagnosis, fused PET/CT images show increased uptake in the esophagus (*arrow in B*) with corresponding wall thickening on CT (*arrow in A*). (*C*) After successful treatment, fused PET/CT images show a normal appearance of the esophagus on CT and PET (*arrow*).

Assessment of splenic involvement has been a clinical and imaging challenge. Staging laparotomy, which is not a rare procedure in patients with HD, revealed splenic involvement in 30% to 40% of cases at presentation [11,30]. The spleen is involved in approximately one fifth of the patients with NHL. Organ size is a poor predictor of lymphomatous involvement. The spleen may be enlarged without being involved, or it may be of normal size despite tumor infiltration. Spleen enlargement has a sensitivity of 38% and a specificity

of 61% for the diagnosis of lymphomatous involvement [13]. The pattern of splenic involvement may be diffuse, more common in HD, or with the appearance of single or multiple small nodules. Involved spleen may appear normal on ultrasound (US) or CT. The reported accuracy of CT for identifying splenic involvement in patients with HD ranges from 37% to 91% when different criteria to suggest splenic involvement have been applied. On MRI, nodular involvement may appear as hypo- or isointense on T1-weighted images and as hyperintense on T2-weighted images and may demonstrate reduced enhancement after administration of gadolinium compared with normal spleen. Splenic involvement may be overlooked in cases in which normal and lymphomatous tissue has similar signal intensity [26,31,32]. On ^{18}F-FDG PET/CT, lymphomatous involvement of the spleen may appear as diffusely increased splenic uptake (although this pattern is not specific and may also

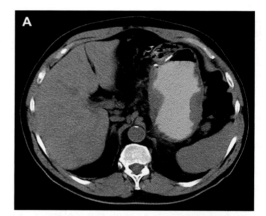

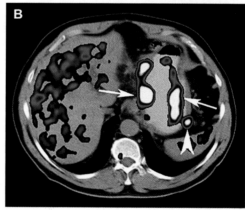

Fig. 2. Gastric lymphoma. CT (*A*) and fused PET/CT (*B*) images show increased ^{18}F-FDG uptake in a primary lymphoma in the stomach (*arrows in B*) and in involved perigastric lymph nodes (*arrowhead in B*). Oral contrast on the CT part of the study allows better delineation of the stomach walls.

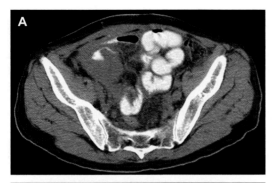

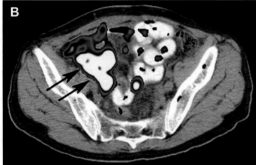

Fig. 3. Intestinal lymphoma. CT (*A*) and fused PET/CT (*B*) images show wall thickening and increased uptake of ^{18}F-FDG in a lesion involving a small bowel loop (*arrows in B*).

be found in nonmalignant "reactive" spleen) and/or focal increased accumulation of the tracer with or without corresponding hypodense lesions on the CT part of the PET/CT study. Comparing the assessment of splenic involvement by ^{18}F-FDG PET and CT in 7 patients with lymphoma, ^{18}F-FDG PET correctly identified or excluded splenic involvement in all patients (accuracy of 100%) as opposed to CT, which was correct for only 4 of the patients (accuracy of 57%) [33]. At times, a splenic mass may be the presenting finding of lymphoma. Metser and coworkers [34] performed PET/CT in 20 patients without a known malignancy who were referred for ^{18}F-FDG PET/CT for characterization of splenic masses. In 10 patients (50%), the lesions were ^{18}F-FDG–avid, and 7 of these patients were diagnosed as having lymphoma. In 5 of these 7 patients, PET also identified nodal disease, whereas 2 patients had lymphoma limited to the spleen, consistent with primary splenic lymphoma.

Liver involvement in lymphoma may present as diffuse disease, as patchy infiltrates originating in the portal areas, as miliary with multiple small lesions, or, less commonly, as large focal lesions [11,35]. The gallbladder, pancreas, peritoneum, adrenal glands, kidneys, female genital organs, and testis are other sites of ENL in the abdomen and pelvis (Fig. 4). Involvement of the gallbladder and

pancreas is almost always secondary to adjacent nodal disease. Because the pancreas has no definable capsule, it may be difficult to distinguish adjacent lymph node disease from pancreatic infiltration. Accurate detection of lymphoma in the pancreas or gallbladder is possible with PET/CT, especially when a mass is detected on the CT part of PET/CT corresponding to PET findings. Involvement of the peritoneum or omentum is found exclusively in NHL, resembling peritoneal involvement by other malignancies, with focal ^{18}F-FDG accumulation in nodules and, often, ascites. Secondary involvement of the adrenal with NHL has been reported to occur in up to 25% of patients during the course of the disease, whereas primary NHL arising from endocrine glands represents only 3% of ENLs. Primary adrenal lymphoma (PAL) is extremely rare. Approximately 70 cases have been reported in the English literature. Because adrenal thickening or an adrenal mass is not an uncommon incidental abnormality on CT, ^{18}F-FDG has been suggested for differentiating

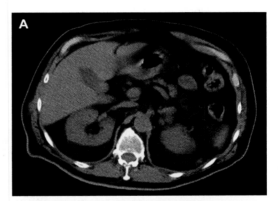

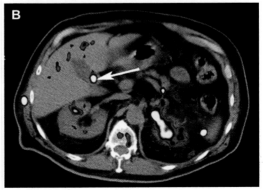

Fig. 4. Lymphoma involving the gallbladder. CT (*A*) and fused PET/CT (*B*) images show a focus of increased ^{18}F-FDG uptake in the gallbladder corresponding to a hyperdense CT lesion (*arrow in B*), demonstrating that the focus seen on PET is attributable to lymphoma involvement and not to physiologic tracer activity in the renal collecting system.

benign incidentaloma from tumoral adrenal involvement [36,37].

Although the incidence of kidney involvement at presentation is only 3%, the kidney is a more common site of recurrence later in the course of NHL. Physiologic ^{18}F-FDG uptake in the renal collecting system may cause false-positive and false-negative PET interpretation of renal involvement in patients with NHL. PET/CT allows for more accurate interpretation, however. Extranodal involvement of the kidney may appear on ^{18}F-FDG PET/CT as multiple focal sites of increased uptake located in the renal cortex, occasionally with corresponding lesions on CT that appear slightly hyperdense on unenhanced and hypodense on contrast-enhanced images; as a contiguous extension from adjacent nodal disease; or, less commonly, in the form of a single mass or diffuse infiltration with organ enlargement [38]. Involvement of HD is rather by invasion of the perirenal space without renal parenchymal involvement [11,35].

Primary lymphomas arising in the female genital organs are rare. They seem to be more common secondary to nodal or extranodal disease (Fig. 5). Based on a report by Kosari and colleagues [39] on 186 patients with lymphoma involving the female genital tract, it seems that the adnexa is the most commonly involved site, followed by the uterine body and cervix, and that the vagina and vulva are the least common sites. The most frequent lymphoma type in the genital tract is DLCL in 45% of cases, followed by Burkitt's lymphoma in 19% of patients. In premenopausal patients, physiologic ^{18}F-FDG uptake may be seen in the ovaries and endometrium during menstruation or in the ovulatory phase of the cycle. It has also been found in association with anticancer therapy–related oligomenorrhea. It is thus important to obtain a full menstrual history when increased ^{18}F-FDG uptake is seen in the genital organs [40]. Lymphoma of the testis accounts for 5% of all testicular malignancies and 1% of all lymphomas. It is the most common testicular malignancy in patients older than 60 years of age, however. Involvement of other mainly extranodal sites at presentation is common, especially such extranodal sites as the contralateral testicle, CNS, skin, and Waldeyer's ring. A high incidence of relapse ranging from 50% to 80% has often been reported in extranodal sites, with the CNS being the relapse site in up to a third of patients. Occasionally, the CNS is the only site of recurrence in patients with testicular lymphoma [41,42]. Although physiologic ^{18}F-FDG uptake is found in the brain cortex and scrotum, disease

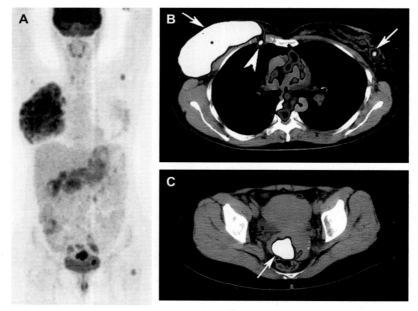

Fig. 5. Burkitt's lymphoma involving the breast and cervix. ^{18}F-FDG PET (maximum intensity projection) (*A*) and fused PET/CT (*B*) images at the level of the thorax demonstrate extensive involvement of the right breast and a smaller site of disease in the left breast (*arrows in B*) as well as involvement of a small right internal mammary lymph node (*arrowhead in B*). (*C*) Fused PET/CT image of the pelvis indicates involvement of the cervix.

involvement may occasionally be identified by the detection of focal sites of a higher intensity compared with that of the background.

Lymphoma of the head and neck

The head and neck region is the second most common site of NHL. Primary ENL of the head and neck may originate in the tonsils, nasopharynx, mandible and/or gingiva, hard palate, parotis, nasal cavity, hypopharynx and larynx, thyroid, ocular adnexa, and paranasal sinuses. Primary head and neck lymphoma accounts for 10% to 20% of all cases of NHL and for 5% of the malignancies in the head and neck region. Most NHLs of the head and neck arise from Waldeyer's ring, including the adenoids and the lymphoid tissue of the nasopharynx and around the pharyngeal opening of the Eustachian tube as well as the oropharynx, involving the palatine tonsils, the lymphoid tissue of the soft palate, and the posterior third or base of the tongue (Fig. 6). Waldeyer's ring is the primary site of NHL in more than 30% of all extranodal sites, most commonly involving the tonsils, followed by the nasopharynx. The tonsil resembles MALT but also has characteristics of peripheral lymph nodes, and the classification of Waldeyer's ring as nodal or extranodal is thus controversial. Lymphoma of the head and neck may be asymptomatic and unsuspected clinically. The nasopharynx was found to be involved in up to 41% of patients when a routine biopsy was performed [43,44].

Reviewing a series of 100 consecutive patients presenting with NHL in the head and neck, Morton and coworkers [45] have reported that otolaryngologic examination performed in patients with cervical nodal disease may reveal unsuspected extranodal disease in Waldeyer's ring in one third of the patients. Lymphoma involving the nasopharynx tends to extend into the airways and tonsils as opposed to carcinoma or sarcoma of the nasopharynx, which tends to extend up into the skull base [44]. Regional nodal involvement, mainly of cervical nodes, is found at presentation or later during the course of the disease in most patients with extranodal involvement of the head and neck [44]. Primary nasal cavity lymphoma is a distinct clinical entity common in Asia, which extends locally into the maxillary and ethmoid sinuses. Lymphoma originating in the paranasal sinuses is aggressive, with frequent distant relapse and early mortality, therefore often warranting CNS prophylaxis.

^{18}F-FDG uptake in the buccal region, nasopharynx, tonsils, and nasal cavity may be physiologic. Even when asymmetric or of high intensity, ^{18}F-FDG uptake does not necessarily indicate the presence of lymphoma and may be related to

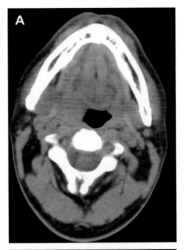

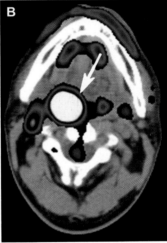

Fig. 6. Head and neck lymphoma. CT (*A*) and fused PET/CT (*B*) images indicate the presence of increased ^{18}F-FDG uptake in the right aspect of the oropharynx (*arrow in B*).

physiologic tracer activity or associated with upper respiratory tract infection (URI). Corresponding CT abnormalities, such as the presence of a soft tissue mass extending into the airways, may assist in the diagnosis of lymphoma on PET/CT, whereas a clinical history of recent URI may help to exclude malignancy as the cause of increased ^{18}F-FDG uptake in this region. In a recent publication by Brianzoni and coworkers [46], the role of PET/CT in radiotherapy planning was assessed in 28 patients, including 4 patients with lymphoma of the head and neck region. PET/CT modified radiotherapy planning in 44% of the study population.

Lymphoma involving the thyroid may present on ^{18}F-FDG PET/CT as a focal abnormality or diffusely increased uptake. Both presentations are, however, nonspecific and may also be seen in goiter, thyroid adenoma, thyroid cancer, or thyroiditis [47]. The most common type of ocular-adnexal lymphoma is MALT lymphoma. Ocular-adnexa lymphoma refers to lymphoma arising in the extraocular orbital space involving the conjunctiva, eyelids, lacrimal gland, and orbital soft tissue [48]. The ability to identify lymphoma in this region on PET/CT may be hampered by the small size of these structures and the physiologic ^{18}F-FDG uptake seen in the ocular muscles and nearby brain cortex. When a distinct mass is identified on the CT part of the PET/CT study, its ^{18}F-FDG avidity can be more easily determined

Lymphoma in the region of the thorax

In the thorax, ENL may involve the lung, pleura, chest wall, myocardium and pericardium, thymus, and breast. In the presence of direct extension from nodal mediastinal disease into the lung or chest wall, HD is staged according to the nodal disease with an associated extranodal (E) designation. These patients have a better prognosis compared with patients with stage IV disease. Pulmonary involvement without nodal disease is more commonly seen in recurrent disease than at presentation. On CT, lymphoma involving the lungs may show variable characteristics. The most common pattern is that of direct extension from nodal disease, whereas other appearances include central ill-defined nodules, rounded or segmental consolidation with an air bronchogram, or nodules or strikes extending peribronchially from the hilum [11,35]. Increased ^{18}F-FDG uptake extending from involved lymph nodes into the lung or in separate pulmonary lesions should lead to the differential diagnosis of lymphomatous lung involvement versus a synchronous primary lung malignancy or a benign condition, such as active granulomatous disease. On PET/CT studies performed after therapy, the presence of ^{18}F-FDG–avid lung abnormalities represents a more difficult diagnostic dilemma, because increased tracer uptake may be related to benign conditions, such as chemotherapy-induced pneumonitis, radiation, opportunistic infections, or bronchiolitis obliterans with organizing pneumonia (BOOP) [3]. Occasionally, the pattern of CT abnormality may be suggestive of infection or treatment-induced abnormalities.

Pleural and pericardial effusions are not uncommon in newly diagnosed lymphoma. Pericardial effusion may be associated mainly with large mediastinal masses. These effusions represent involvement of the pleura or pericardium by lymphoma or may be of a reactive etiology. Pleural involvement may manifest as plaques, discrete nodules,

or a combination of the two, or it may be underappreciated on CT when interpreted alone but may be identified on fused ^{18}F-FDG PET/CT images when corresponding in location to PET abnormalities (Fig. 7) [49].

The most common type of chest wall involvement is by direct extension from nodal disease in the anterior mediastinum. Chest wall involvement has been documented in 6% of patients with HD. Detection of chest wall invasion is of clinical relevance because it is associated with higher relapse rates and requires more aggressive therapy [11]. The fused PET/CT data allow for improved identification of chest wall invasion by precise localization of the extent of the mediastinal PET abnormality. In patients with HD, the thymus is considered "nodal," and thymic involvement thus does not change the stage of the disease. Up to half of the patients with thoracic HD may show an enlarged thymus, which may be persistent after successful treatment as a result of rebound thymic hyperplasia or the development of thymic cysts. Active disease and benign thymic hyperplasia may be associated with ^{18}F-FDG accumulation. The timing relative to

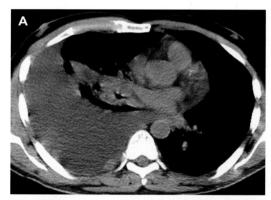

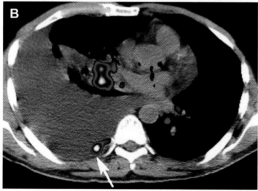

Fig. 7. Lymphoma involving the pleura. CT (*A*) and fused PET/CT (*B*) images show increased ^{18}F-FDG uptake in a pleural plaque (*arrow in B*), suggesting the malignant etiology of the pleural effusion.

therapy and evidence or absence of active disease elsewhere in the body may assist in differentiating the two conditions. When the etiology is uncertain, a biopsy may be indicated [50].

Primary lymphoma of the breast is rare, accounting for less than 2% of ENLs and 0.38% to 0.7% of all cases of NHL. Breast NHL represents 0.14% of all female breast malignancies [1]. Secondary breast lymphoma is also rare but represents the largest group of metastatic mammary tumors [51]. The most common type of unilateral breast lymphoma is DLCL, accounting for 45% to 79% of the cases. Less common is Burkitt's lymphoma, which may present as rapidly disseminating bilateral diffuse disease mainly affecting puerperal women (see Fig. 5). MALT lymphoma of the breast is a subgroup with a relative frequency of 0% to 75% [1,51]. The radiographic and mammographic features of breast lymphoma are nonspecific. Breast density, which poses difficulties in interpretation of mammography, does not seem to affect the accuracy of PET in identifying lesions in the breast [52]. In addition, the whole-body imaging capability of PET enables detection of unexpected involvement of the breast, because mammography is not performed routinely in lymphoma staging and CT is not accurate for assessment of breast pathologic findings.

Lymphoma involving the bone marrow and cortical bone

Involvement of the bone marrow is found in approximately 50% to 80% of low-grade NHL, 25% to 40% of high-grade NHL, and 5% to 14% of HD at diagnosis, with a further increase in incidence later in the course of the disease. Bone marrow involvement signifies advanced-stage disease and may affect treatment and prognosis. Pakos and colleagues [53] performed a meta-analysis of the literature on the issue of the ability of ^{18}F-FDG PET to evaluate bone marrow infiltration in the staging of lymphoma. Thirteen studies with a total of 587 patients were analyzed. Bone marrow biopsy (BMB) had a sensitivity and specificity of 51% and 91%, respectively, when compared with PET. In some patients, however, PET results that were considered to be false-positive findings initially because of negative BMB marrow turned out to be true-positive findings when involvement was confirmed on repeat biopsy to sites guided by PET findings (Fig. 8). PET had a better sensitivity in HD and in aggressive types of NHL compared with less aggressive NHL. Before therapy, a pattern of patchy increased marrow uptake is suggestive of lymphomatous involvement, whereas diffuse uptake, mainly in HD, may be associated with reactive hematopoietic changes within the marrow or myeloid hyperplasia [54]. Because neither bone marrow biopsy nor ^{18}F-FDG PET imaging or MRI is highly reliable as a single technique, Kostakoglu and coworkers [3] suggested their complementary use for assessment of marrow involvement in lymphoma.

After treatment, mainly chemotherapy, or after granulocyte colony-stimulating factor (G-CSF), increased reactive ^{18}F-FDG bone marrow uptake is often detected and is difficult to differentiate from active marrow disease [55]. Increased splenic ^{18}F-FDG uptake, which often accompanies skeletal uptake after G-CSF therapy, was suggested to represent a "clue" for correct diagnosis [56].

Primary bone involvement occurs in 3% to 5% of patients with NHL, and 25% of patients with NHL have secondary bone involvement. Primary bone involvement is rare in HD (1%–4% at presentation). Secondary bone involvement occurs in 5% to 20% of patients with HD during the course of the disease, however [11,57]. Moog and coworkers [58] have reported ^{18}F-FDG PET to be more sensitive and specific than ^{99m}Tc-methylene diphosphonate (MDP) bone scintigraphy for the detection of osseous involvement of lymphoma. Detection of malignant bone involvement on CT depends on the presence of a considerable amount of bone destruction. Early lymphomatous bone involvement may thus show positive lesions on PET that have a normal CT appearance [11].

Lymphoma involving the nervous system

Lymphoma of the CNS is confined to the cranial-spinal axis, including the brain, eye, leptomeninges,

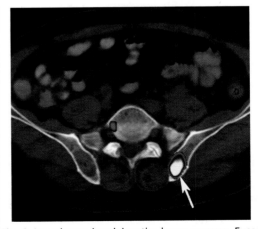

Fig. 8. Lymphoma involving the bone marrow. Fused PET/CT images show increased ^{18}F-FDG uptake in the posterior aspect of the left ileum. PET/CT-guided bone marrow biopsy was positive for lymphomatous involvement (*arrow*).

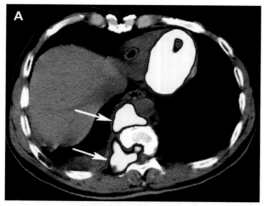

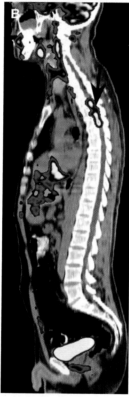

Fig. 9. Lymphoma involving the nervous system. Fused PET/CT transaxial image (*A*) illustrate extension of lymphoma from the paravertebral space through the intervertebral neural foramina (*arrow in A*). Fused PET/CT sagittal image (*B*) illustrates spinal involvement in a patient who presented with abrupt spinal cord compression (*arrow in B*).

and spinal cord, and accounts for 1% to 4% of malignant brain tumors and 2% to 4% of ENLs [1]. The incidence of CNS lymphoma is increasing in immunocompromised and immunocompetent patients [59]. The brain and meninges are the most commonly affected sites, followed by deep structures of the brain, including the periventricular

areas, corpus callosum, basal ganglia, brain stem, and cerebellum. Most CNS lymphomas in immunocompetent patients are of the DLCL subtype. Patients with lymphoblastic or Burkitt's lymphoma carry a 25% risk of CNS relapse. A high incidence of CNS relapse was also reported in association with high-grade lymphomas located in the testicles and paranasal sinuses [60,61].

Spinal cord compression may be the initial manifestation of lymphoma caused by localized ENL, or more commonly, by an epidural mass developing as an extension from involved nodes through the intervertebral neural foramina [62]. A valuable contribution of the CT portion of the PET/CT study in lymphoma is its capacity to identify the presence of the increased uptake in epidural masses and neural foramen invasion that may accompany vertebral or paravertebral disease (Fig. 9) [63].

Detection of lymphoma of the brain cortex may be hampered by the presence of physiologic ^{18}F-FDG uptake. The latter may be less of a burden for detection of lesions in deeper brain structures. Palmedo and coworkers [59] compared the role of ^{18}F-FDG PET with MRI in immunocompetent patients with biopsy-proven CNS lymphoma. PET identified lymphomatous lesions in six of seven patients and missed a 4-mm lesion in a single patient. During follow-up, PET accurately identified recurrence in three patients and excluded disease in five patients, with three of these patients having false-positive findings on an MRI study. A negative PET scan early during therapy was a reliable predictor of complete remission. It should be mentioned that steroid therapy, which is often initiated when brain involvement is suspected, may cause a reduction in ^{18}F-FDG accumulation and lead to false-negative findings.

Peripheral neuropathy in patients with lymphoma may be caused by drug neurotoxicity, infection, nerve root compression, postradiation neuropathy, vasculitis, or infiltration of the peripheral nerve system (neurolymphomatosis). Two recently published case reports illustrated the benefit of ^{18}F-FDG PET/CT imaging in the detection (sometimes the first modality to suggest the diagnosis) and monitoring response to therapy of neurolymphomatosis [64,65].

Summary

Lymphoma may originate in extranodal sites. ENL may also be secondary to and accompany nodal disease. ENL is probably more common than previously thought, with an incidence of approximately 25% in the overall population of patients with lymphoma, which may be even higher in some specific subtypes, such as MALT. ^{18}F-FDG imaging has an essential role in the staging of lymphoma, in monitoring the response to therapy, and in detection of recurrence. The introduction of ^{18}F-FDG PET/CT hybrid imaging allows for accurate localization of disease and may be specifically beneficial for the detection of unexpected extranodal sites of disease or exclusion of disease in the presence of nonspecific extranodal CT findings. Accurate staging and localization often dictate the appropriate treatment strategy in patients with lymphoma. Therefore, at any stage in the course of the disease, the potential presence of extranodal disease should be considered when interpreting ^{18}F-FDG PET/CT studies in patients with NHL and HD.

References

[1] Zucca E, Conconi A, Cavalli F. Treatment of extranodal lymphomas. Best Pract Res Clin Haematol 2002;15:533–47.

[2] Glass AG, Karnell LH, Menck HR. The National Cancer Data Base report on non Hodgkin's lymphoma. Cancer 1997;80:2311–20.

[3] Kostakoglu L, Goldsmith SJ. Fluorine-18 fluorodeoxyglucose positron emission tomography in the staging and follow-up of lymphoma: is it time to shift gears? Eur J Nucl Med 2000;27:1564–78.

[4] Hasenclever D, Diehl V. A prognostic score for advanced Hodgkin's disease. International Prognostic Factors Project on Advanced Hodgkin's Disease. N Engl J Med 1998;339:1506–14.

[5] Groves FD, Linet MS, Travis LB, et al. Cancer surveillance series: non-Hodgkin's lymphoma incidence by histologic subtype in the United States from 1978 through 1995. J Natl Cancer Inst 2000;92:1240–51.

[6] Economopoulos T, Asprou N, Stathakis N, et al. Primary extranodal non-Hodgkin's lymphoma in adults: clinicopathological and survival characteristics. Leuk Lymphoma 1996;21:131–6.

[7] Cavalli F, Isaacson PG, Gascoyne R, et al. MALT lymphomas. Hematology (Am Soc Hematol Educ Program) 2001;1:241–58.

[8] Maes B, De Wolf-Peeters C. Marginal zone cell lymphoma—an update on recent advances. Histopathology 2002;40:117–26.

[9] Leonard JP, Schattner EJ, Coleman M. Biology and management of mantle cell lymphoma. Curr Opin Oncol 2001;13:342–7.

[10] Samaha H, Dumontet C, Ketterer N, et al. Mantle cell lymphoma: a retrospective study of 121 cases. Leukemia 1998;12:1281–7.

[11] Guermazi A, Brice P, de Kerviler EE, et al. Extranodal Hodgkin disease: spectrum of disease. Radiographics 2001;21:161–79.

[12] Isasi CR, Lu P, Blaufox MD. A metaanalysis of 18F-2-deoxy-2-fluoro-D-glucose positron emission tomography in the staging and restaging of patients with lymphoma. Cancer 2005;104:1066–74.

[13] Moog F, Bangerter M, Diederichs CG, et al. Extranodal malignant lymphoma: detection with FDG PET versus CT. Radiology 1998;206:475–81.

[14] Israel O, Keidar Z, Bar-Shalom R. Positron emission tomography in the evaluation of lymphoma. Semin Nucl Med 2004;34:166–79.

[15] Wiedmann E, Baican B, Hertel A, et al. Positron emission tomography (PET) for staging and evaluation of response to treatment in patients with Hodgkin's disease. Leuk Lymphoma 1999;34:545–51.

[16] Raanani P, Shasha Y, Perry C, et al. Is CT scan still necessary for staging in Hodgkin and non-Hodgkin lymphoma patients in the PET/CT era? Ann Oncol 2006;17(1):117–22.

[17] Rodriguez M, Ahlstrom H, Sundin A, et al. [18F] FDG PET in gastric non-Hodgkin's lymphoma. Acta Oncol 1997;36:577–84.

[18] Schaefer NG, Hany TF, Taverna C, et al. Non-Hodgkin lymphoma and Hodgkin disease: coregistered FDG PET and CT at staging and restaging—do we need contrast-enhanced CT? Radiology 2004;232:823–9.

[19] Bertoni F, Zucca E. State-of-the-art therapeutics: marginal-zone lymphoma. J Clin Oncol 2005;23:6415–20.

[20] Nakamura S, Aoyagi K, Furuse M, et al. B-cell monoclonality precedes the development of gastric MALT lymphoma in Helicobacter pylori-associated chronic gastritis. Am J Pathol 1998;152:1271–9.

[21] Hoffmann M, Kletter K, Becherer A, et al. 18F-fluorodeoxyglucose positron emission tomography (18F-FDG-PET) for staging and follow-up of marginal zone B-cell lymphoma. Oncology 2003;64:336–40.

[22] Beal KP, Yeung HW, Yahalom J. FDG-PET scanning for detection and staging of extranodal marginal zone lymphomas of the MALT type: a report of 42 cases. Ann Oncol 2005;16(3):473–8.

[23] Natsag J, Tomiyama N, Inoue A, et al. Pulmonary mucosa-associated lymphoid tissue type lymphoma with increased accumulation of fluorine 18-fluorodeoxyglucose on positron emission tomography. J Comput Assist Tomogr 2005;29:640–3.

[24] d'Amore F, Brincker H, Gronbaek K, et al. Non-Hodgkin's lymphoma of the gastrointestinal tract: a population-based analysis of incidence, geographic distribution, clinicopathologic presentation features, and prognosis. Danish Lymphoma Study Group. J Clin Oncol 1994;12:1673–84.

[25] Salvagno L, Soraru M, Busetto M, et al. Gastric non-Hodgkin's lymphoma: analysis of 252 patients from a multicenter study. Tumori 1999;85:113–21.

[26] Kumar R, Xiu Y, Potenta S, et al. 18F-FDG PET for evaluation of the treatment response in

patients with gastrointestinal tract lymphomas. J Nucl Med 2004;45:1796–803.

[27] Poggi MM, Cong PJ, Coleman CN, et al. Low-grade follicular lymphoma of the small intestine. J Clin Gastroenterol 2002;34:155–9.

[28] Metser U, Goor O, Lerman H, et al. PET-CT of extranodal lymphoma. AJR Am J Roentgenol 2004; 182:1579–86.

[29] Wahl RL. Why nearly all PET of abdominal and pelvic cancers will be performed as PET/CT. J Nucl Med 2004;45(Suppl 1):82S–95S.

[30] Shirkhoda A, Ros PR, Farah J, et al. Lymphoma of the solid abdominal viscera. Radiol Clin North Am 1990;28:785–99.

[31] Urba WJ, Longo DL. Hodgkin's disease. N Engl J Med 1992;326:678–87.

[32] Munker R, Stengel A, Stabler A, et al. Diagnostic accuracy of ultrasound and computed tomography in the staging of Hodgkin's disease. Cancer 1995;76(8):1460–6.

[33] Rini JN, Leonidas JC, Tomas MB, et al. 18F-FDG PET versus CT for evaluating the spleen during initial staging of lymphoma. J Nucl Med 2003; 44:1072–4.

[34] Metser U, Miller E, Kessler A, et al. Solid splenic masses: evaluation with 18F-FDG PET/CT. J Nucl Med 2005;46:52–9.

[35] Fishman EK, Kuhlman JE, Jones RJ. CT of lymphoma: spectrum of disease. Radiographics 1991;11:647–69.

[36] Kumar R, Xiu Y, Mavi A, et al. FDG-PET imaging in primary bilateral adrenal lymphoma: a case report and review of the literature. Clin Nucl Med 2005;30:222–30.

[37] Metser U, Miller E, Lerman H, et al. 18F-fluoro-deoxyglucose-PET/CT in the evaluation of adrenal masses. J Nucl Med 2006;47:32–7.

[38] Charnsangavej C. Lymphoma of the genitourinary tract. Radiol Clin North Am 1990;28:865–77.

[39] Kosari F, Daneshbod Y, Parwaresch R, et al. Lymphomas of the female genital tract: a study of 186 cases and review of the literature. Am J Surg Pathol 2005;29:1512–20.

[40] Lerman H, Metser U, Grisaru D, et al. Normal and abnormal 18F-FDG endometrial and ovarian uptake in pre- and postmenopausal patients: assessment by PET/CT. J Nucl Med 2005;45:266–71.

[41] Tondini C, Ferreri AJ, Siracusano L, et al. Diffuse large-cell lymphoma of the testis. J Clin Oncol 1999;17:2854–8.

[42] Fonseca R, Habermann TM, Colgan JP, et al. Testicular lymphoma is associated with a high incidence of extranodal recurrence. Cancer 2000;88: 154–61.

[43] Tan LH. Lymphomas involving Waldeyer's ring: placement, paradigms, peculiarities, pitfalls, patterns and postulates. Ann Acad Med Singapore 2004;33(Suppl 4):15–26.

[44] King AD, Lei KI, Richards PS, et al. Non-Hodgkin's lymphoma of the nasopharynx: CT and MR imaging. Clin Radiol 2003;58:621–5.

[45] Morton RP, Sillars HA, Benjamin CS. Incidence of 'unsuspected' extranodal head and neck lymphoma. Clin Otolaryngol Allied Sci 1992;17: 373–5.

[46] Brianzoni E, Rossi G, Ancidei S, et al. Radiotherapy planning: PET/CT scanner performances in the definition of gross tumour volume and clinical target volume. Eur J Nucl Med Mol Imaging 2005;32:1392–9.

[47] Cohen MS, Arslan N, Dehdashti F, et al. Risk of malignancy in thyroid incidentalomas identified by fluorodeoxyglucose-positron emission tomography. Surgery 2001;130:941–6.

[48] Uno T, Isobe K, Shikama N, Nishikawa A, et al. Radiotherapy for extranodal, marginal zone, B-cell lymphoma of mucosa-associated lymphoid tissue originating in the ocular adnexa: a multiinstitutional, retrospective review of 50 patients. Cancer 2003;98:865–71.

[49] Toaff JS, Metser U, Gottfried M, et al. Differentiation between malignant and benign pleural effusion in patients with extra-pleural primary malignancies: assessment with positron emission tomography-computed tomography. Invest Radiol 2005;40:204–9.

[50] Ferdinand B, Gupta P, Kramer EL. Spectrum of thymic uptake at 18F-FDG PET. Radiographics 2004;24:1611–6.

[51] Topalovski M, Crisan D, Mattson JC. Lymphoma of the breast. A clinicopathologic study of primary and secondary cases. Arch Pathol Lab Med 1999;123:1208–18.

[52] Kumar R, Xiu Y, Dhurairaj T, et al. F-18 FDG positron emission tomography in non-Hodgkin lymphoma of the breast. Clin Nucl Med 2005; 30:246–8.

[53] Pakos EE, Fotopoulos AD, Ioannidis JP. 18F-FDG PET for evaluation of bone marrow infiltration in staging of lymphoma: a meta-analysis. J Nucl Med 2005;46:958–63.

[54] Carr R, Barrington SF, Madan B, et al. Detection of lymphoma in bone marrow by whole-body positron emission tomography. Blood 1998;91: 3340–6.

[55] Kazama T, Faria SC, Varavithya V, et al. FDG PET in the evaluation of treatment for lymphoma: clinical usefulness and pitfalls. Radiographics 2005;25:191–207.

[56] Sugawara Y, Zasadny KR, Kison PV, et al. Splenic fluorodeoxyglucose uptake increased by granulocyte colony-stimulating factor therapy: PET imaging results. J Nucl Med 1999;40:1456–62.

[57] Burkes BJ, Gospodarowicz M. Primary non-Hodgkin's lymphoma of bone. Semin Oncol 1999;26:270–5.

[58] Moog F, Kotzerke J, Reske SN. FDG PET can replace bone scintigraphy in primary staging of malignant lymphoma. J Nucl Med 1999;40: 1407–13.

[59] Palmedo H, Urbach H, Bender H, et al. FDG-PET in immunocompetent patients with primary central nervous system lymphoma:

correlation with MRI and clinical follow-up. Eur J Nucl Med Mol Imaging 2006;33(2): 164–8.

[60] Ferreri AJ, Abrey LE, Blay JY, et al. Summary statement on primary central nervous system lymphomas from the Eighth International Conference on Malignant Lymphoma, Lugano, Switzerland, 2002. J Clin Oncol 2003;21: 2407–14.

[61] Hollender A, Kvaloy S, Nome O, et al. Central nervous system involvement following diagnosis of non-Hodgkin's lymphoma: a risk model. Ann Oncol 2002;13:1099–107.

[62] Pels H, Vogt I, Klockgether T, et al. Primary non-Hodgkin's lymphoma of the spinal cord. Spine 2000;25:2262–4.

[63] Metser U, Lerman H, Blank A, et al. Malignant involvement of the spine: assessment by 18F-FDG PET/CT. J Nucl Med 2004;45:279–84.

[64] Kanter P, Zeidman A, Streifler J, et al. PET-CT imaging of combined brachial and lumbosacral neurolymphomatosis. Eur J Haematol 2005;74:66–9.

[65] Bokstein F, Goor O, Shihman B, et al. Assessment of neurolymphomatosis by brachial plexus biopsy and PET/CT. Report of a case. J Neurooncol 2005;72:163–7.

RADIOLOGIC
CLINICS
OF NORTH AMERICA

Radiol Clin N Am 45 (2007) 711–718

Critical Role of 18F-Labeled Fluorodeoxyglucose PET in the Management of Patients with Arthroplasty

Hongming Zhuang, MD, PhD[a,b], Hua Yang, MD[a], Abass Alavi, MD[a,*]

- Accuracy of 18F-labeled fluorodeoxyglucose PET in the evaluation of infection associated with arthroplasty with a dedicated full-ring PET scanner
- Potential sources of suboptimal results for fluorodeoxyglucose PET imaging in painful arthroplasty

- *Coincident camera*
- *Combined PET and CT*
- Evaluating bone allograft after hip revision arthroplasty
- Summary
- References

The success of arthroplasty has greatly improved the quality of life for many patients with degenerative, arthritic, or injured joints. Some patients develop persistent pain at the site of arthroplasty after surgery, however. In most patients, the pain is caused by biomechanical failure (loosening), whereas in a small number of such patients, it is attributable to periprosthetic infection [1–5]. One of the most difficult diagnostic challenges in patients with painful prostheses is how to distinguish between aseptic mechanical loosening and periprosthetic infection. Most periprosthetic infections remain undiagnosed before revision surgery is undertaken. Clinically, these two clinical entities have similar presentations. The current tests to establish the diagnosis of infection before surgery include routine radiography, bacterial culture after joint aspiration, three-phase bone scan, gallium scan, and labeled leukocyte scintigraphy. Results from these tests are suboptimal, however, because of high rates of false-positive and false-negative findings. Accurate diagnosis or exclusion of infection is critical before revision surgery. Treatment of aseptic loosening requires a single revision operation, whereas patients with infection require a long period of treatment before surgery is contemplated. Currently, multiple tests are used for differentiating aseptic loosening from infection. A white

This article was previously published in PET Clinics 2006;1:99–106.
This article is partially supported by an N14 grant 5R01AR048241 (to AA).
a Division of Nuclear Medicine, Department of Radiology, University of Pennsylvania School of Medicine, Hospital of the University of Pennsylvania, 110 Donner Building, 3400 Spruce Street, Philadelphia, PA 19104, USA
b Division of Nuclear Medicine, Department of Radiology, University of Pennsylvania School of Medicine, The Children's Hospital of Philadelphia, 34th Street and Civic Center Boulevard, Philadelphia, PA 19104, USA
* Corresponding author.
E-mail address: abass.alavi@uphs.upenn.edu (A. Alavi).

doi:10.1016/j.rcl.2007.05.010

blood cell count, erythrocyte sedimentation rate, and C-reactive protein level are all frequently performed for this purpose but provide nonspecific results. Plain films have a limited role in such clinical settings, because infection and loosening have similar findings. Aspiration biopsy, if positive, can confirm infection before surgery. A negative joint aspiration result cannot exclude the diagnosis of infection [6], however, especially in patients who have received antibiotic therapy before aspiration biopsy [7,8]. Bone and gallium scintigraphy was initially used in the evaluation of infection after arthroplasty. Most infections cannot be diagnosed accurately by bone and gallium scans, however [9]. Although three-phase bone scintigraphy has been used in the evaluation of painful prosthesis replacement, it lacks adequate accuracy [10]. Indium 111–labeled leukocyte scintigraphy, when combined with technetium (Tc)-99m–sulfur colloid bone marrow imaging, may provide reasonable accuracy for the detection of infection after arthroplasty [11–14]. This technique requires separating, labeling, and reinjection of the patient's white blood cells, however, which is quite complex and time-consuming and increases the chance of iatrogenic errors [15]. In addition, 24-hour delayed imaging is necessary before a diagnosis can be made, which further adds to the complexity of the procedure.

In recent years, 18F-labeled fluorodeoxyglucose (FDG) PET has been used successfully for assessing a multitude of malignant disorders. FDG is specific for neoplastic tumor, however, and it also accumulates at the sites of infection and inflammation [16–23]. As a result of these observations, FDG-PET has emerged as a promising imaging modality for the evaluation of a variety of infectious and inflammatory processes [24,25], including those of the musculoskeletal system [26–36]. There are reports indicating that FDG-PET is more accurate

than conventional nuclear medicine procedures in the evaluation of inflammation or infection [37–39]. In addition to providing high-quality images within a reasonably short time, FDG-PET scan results are not adversely affected by a metal prosthesis [40]. Therefore, FDG-PET is emerging as an important imaging modality in the evaluation of arthroplasty-associated complications.

Accuracy of 18F-labeled fluorodeoxyglucose PET in the evaluation of infection associated with arthroplasty with a dedicated full-ring PET scanner

The accuracy of FDG-PET from the pooled data of the major publications in the English literature is 90.4% (range: 68.6%–100%) for assessing painful hip prostheses and 83.1% (range: 77.8%–100%) for knee prostheses [Table 1]. In general, most publications demonstrate that for the evaluation of possible hip prosthesis infection, the specificity of FDG-PET is slightly higher than its sensitivity. In contrast, FDG-PET has high sensitivity but moderate specificity for examining painful knee prostheses for infection [see Table 1].

The largest sample of patients with hip prostheses examined with FDG-PET was reported in a recent publication by Reinartz and colleagues [10]. In this study, these investigators recruited 63 patients with 92 hip prostheses with possible periprosthetic infection. They noted that the sensitivity, specificity, and accuracy of FDG-PET were 93.9%, 94.9%, and 94.6%, respectively. These results are in contrast to the results of three-phase bone scintigraphy, which achieved sensitivity, specificity, and accuracy of 68%, 76%, and 74%, respectively. The authors concluded that FDG-PET is a highly accurate diagnostic procedure that is able to differentiate reliably between aseptic loosening and periprosthetic

Table 1: **Accuracy of 18F-labeled fluorodeoxyglucose imaging of painful prostheses using a full-ring dedicated PET scanner**

Type	Authors [reference]	Year	No. prostheses	Sensitivity	Specificity	Accuracy
Hip	Manthey et al [55]	2002	14	100% (3/3)	100% (11/11)	100% (14/14)
	Vanquickenborne et al [43]	2003	17	87.5% (7/8)	77.8% (7/9)	82.4% (14/17)
	Stumpe et al [44]	2004	35	33.3% (3/9)	80.8% (21/26)	68.6% (24/35)
	Reddy et al [42]	2005	81	91.3% (21/23)	96.5% (56/58)	95.1% (77/81)
	Reinartz et al [10]	2005	92	93.9% (31/33)	94.9% (56/59)	94.6% (87/92)
Hip total			239	85.5% (65/76)	92.6% (151/163)	90.4% (216/239)
Knee	Van Acker et al [53]	2001	21	100 (6/6)	73.3 (11/15)	81.0% (17/21)
	Zhuang et al [41]	2001	36	90.9% (10/11)	72.0% (18/25)	77.8% (28/36)
	Manthey et al [55]	2002	14	100% (1/1)	100% (13/13)	100% (14/14)
Knee Total			71	94.4% (17/18)	79.2% (42/53)	83.1% (59/71)

infection [10]. The results of this investigation are similar to those of our group. In an early investigation by our group involving 62 patients and 74 lower extremity prostheses (36 knee and 38 hip prostheses), FDG-PET demonstrated an overall sensitivity of 90.5% and specificity of 81.1% in the diagnosis of periprosthetic infection [41]. The sensitivity, specificity, and accuracy of PET for detecting infection associated with 38 hip arthroplasties were 90%, 89.3%, and 89.5%, respectively [41]. In our group's recent data on 81 painful hip prostheses, FDG-PET correctly diagnosed 21 of the 23 infected cases, with a sensitivity of 91.3%. The results of FDG-PET were positive only in 2 of the 58 aseptic prostheses, with a specificity of 96.5%. FDG-PET imaging demonstrated a positive predictive value of 91.3% and a negative predictive value of 96.6%. The overall accuracy of FDG-PET in this clinical setting is 95.1% [42]. In certain studies with a small sample of patients, however, relatively low rates of accurate results have been reported. For example, in an investigation involving 17 hip prostheses, Vanquickenborne and coworkers [43] found that FDG-PET had a sensitivity of 87.5%, a specificity of 77.8%, and an accuracy of 82.4%. These results seem suboptimal compared with those of single photon emission computed tomography (SPECT) images with ^{99m}Tc-hexamethylpropylene-amine oxime (HMPAO)-labeled leukocyte scintigraphy. The least accurate result was reported by Stumpe and colleagues [44] when they showed that FDG-PET only has an accuracy of 68.6%.

Several factors might account for the discrepant results reported by the different groups. The first and probably most important answer for this variance is the lack of uniform criteria used for the diagnosis of periprosthetic infection. By now, it is well known that there is frequently nonspecific FDG uptake after hip arthroplasty, which can last as long as 2 decades in patients without any complications [45]. The nonspecific FDG activity is usually around the head and neck portion of the prosthesis [Fig. 1]. The nonspecific activity around the neck portion of the hip prosthesis is probably caused by the accumulation of macrophages and multinuclear giant cells attributable to polyethylene wear particles [46–48]. Therefore, caution should be exercised in interpreting FDG activity in these locations so as to minimize the number of false-positive results. In addition, the sites of the increased FDG accumulation seem to be more important than the intensity of the FDG uptake at these locations [49]. Vanquickenborne and colleagues [43] interpreted PET images to represent infection when FDG uptake around the prosthesis is two scores higher than that in the contralateral distal femur. In contrast, Reinartz and his coworkers [10,50] considered infection

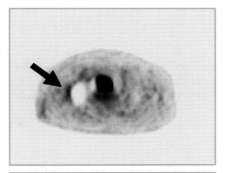

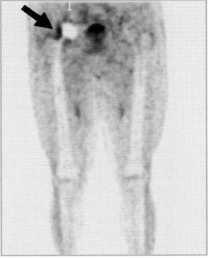

Fig. 1. Transaxial (*upper*) and coronal (*lower*) views of FDG-PET images of an asymptomatic patient with a history of right hip arthroplasty. Arrows point to the nonspecific FDG uptake in the neck region of the prosthesis.

as the diagnosis when increased FDG activity in the periprosthetic soft tissue and arthroplasty interface was observed. Our group [49,51] has used similar criteria for infection as those of Reinartz and his coworkers [10,50]. We think that the abnormal FDG uptake along the prosthesis-bone interface in the middle portion of the shaft of the prosthesis is the most reliable indicator of periprosthetic infection [Fig. 2]. The degree of FDG uptake alone can be misleading, because there is a significant overlap between aseptic loosening and periprosthetic infection with regard to the intensity of the activity noted on these scans [10]. In an investigation by Reinartz and colleagues [10] involving a total of 92 hip prostheses, the average standardized uptake value was 5.3 ± 2.7 for periprosthetic infection, which was not significantly different ($P = .35$) from that (5.0 ± 3.0) of aseptic loosening. This might explain why Vanquickenborne and coworkers [43] reported slightly less accurate results compared with those of

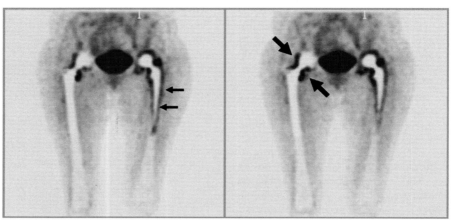

Fig. 2. A 59-year-old man with bilateral hip arthroplasty and pain on the left side. FDG-PET images revealed intense activity in the region of the neck of the right hip prosthesis (*large arrows*), which was interpreted to be a nonspecific finding and not representing infection. FDG-PET also demonstrated diffuse activity along the middle portion of the shaft of the left hip prosthesis (*small arrows*), which was considered strongly suggestive of periprosthetic infection. The periprosthetic infection was confirmed by subsequent surgery.

the Reinartz and colleagues [10], because intensity of the activity was considered the major criterion used by former group for diagnosing periprosthetic infection. In addition to different diagnostic criteria used by different groups, standards by which the presence of or lack of infection was confirmed and the composition of the patient population recruited, which included subjects with different prevalence of the disease, might also have contributed to the differences in the accuracy of the results reported by different investigators.

The experience with FDG-PET in the evaluation of knee prostheses is considerably less than that in hip prostheses. The accuracy of FDG-PET in the evaluation of knee prostheses is somewhat lower than that in hip prostheses [41] for unclear reasons. Capsulitis or synovitis attributable to the loosening of the knee prosthesis can result in intense FDG activity [52,53] that is difficult to distinguish from the hypermetabolism caused by infection. In addition, it has been proposed that attenuation correction-induced artifact around a knee prosthesis might render the interpretation difficult [54]. Van Acker and coworkers [53] assessed the potential of FDG-PET in a group of 21 patients with painful knee prostheses. Using focal FDG uptake at the bone-prosthesis interface as the criterion for infection, they found that the sensitivity, specificity, and positive predictive value of FDG-PET were 100%, 73%, and 60%, respectively, in the diagnosis of periprosthetic knee infection. Similarly, in a study involving 36 knee prostheses, the sensitivity, specificity, and positive predictive value of FDG-PET were shown to be 90.9%, 72.0%, and 58.8%, respectively [41]. In an investigation involving 14

painful knee prostheses evaluated by FDG-PET, however, Manthey and colleagues [55] were able to exclude infection in all the noninfected patients with sensitivity, specificity, and positive predictive values of 100%, 100%, and 100%, respectively. The number of patients in this investigation is relatively small; therefore, the results cannot be generalized to the overall patient population referred for this examination. Also, similar to what was described for hip prostheses, different diagnostic criteria used by different groups could have contributed to the difference in the accuracy of the results reported by different groups.

Potential sources of suboptimal results for fluorodeoxyglucose PET imaging in painful arthroplasty

Coincident camera

It is important to note that evaluation of a painful prosthesis by a coincidence PET camera is likely to provide unsatisfactory results. Love and coworkers [56] studied FDG uptake in 40 hip and 19 knee prostheses using a coincidence detection system. They noted that regardless of the how the images were interpreted, the accuracy of this approach is suboptimal. The best accuracy by using the most favorable schemes was 71% (78% for hip prostheses and 58% for knee prostheses). In contrast, the accuracy of the combined leukocyte and bone marrow imaging was 95% in their study population. Therefore, the authors concluded that the coincidence detection system is less accurate than combined labeled leukocyte and bone marrow

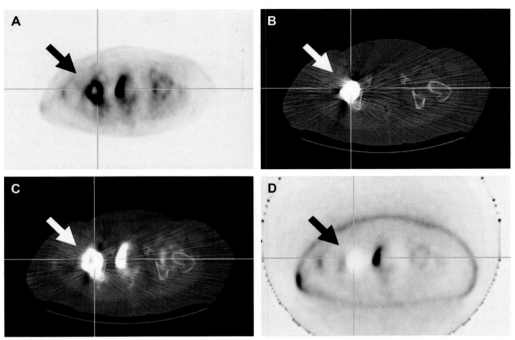

Fig. 3. PET-CT images from a patient with a right hip prosthesis. The attenuation-corrected image (*A*) demon-strated intense activity (*black arrow*) corresponding to the metal prosthesis on CT (*B*) and fused PET-CT (*C*) images (*white arrows*). This intense activity is an artifact caused by CT for reconstructing attenuation correc-tion imaging. (*D*) Non-attenuation-corrected image is negative in the corresponding region (*black arrow*).

imaging for diagnosing infection of the failed pros-thetic joint [56].

Combined PET and CT

The combined PET and CT instruments have certain advantages over PET alone in the evaluation of a variety of malignancies. Nevertheless, it is impor-tant to note that in contrast to conventional PET scanners, when a cesium (Cs)-137 or Germanium-68 (Ge-68) source is used for attenuation correction and is not significantly affected by metal [40,57,58], the CT-corrected images often have significant arti-fact at the location of the prosthesis, which inter-feres with the optimal interpretation of the result generated [Fig. 3] [59,60]. Therefore, when PET-CT is used for the evaluation of a painful prosthesis, non-attenuation-corrected images must be inter-preted for this purpose so as to avoid false-positive results.

Evaluating bone allograft after hip revision arthroplasty

Bone loss with or without evidence of aseptic loos-ening or periprosthetic infection is a long-term complication after total hip arthroplasty [61]. It occurs with all types of materials and in almost all prosthetic systems. Revision total hip arthroplasty

often presents surgeons with the difficult task of restoring bone loss at the site [62]. Therefore, the use of bone allograft in revision hip arthroplasty has gained acceptance [62–65]. Monitoring the incorporation and vitality of bone allograft is diffi-cult by conventional imaging methods, however [66,67]. CT and MRI usually do not play a signifi-cant role in such clinical settings because of artifacts induced by the metal prosthesis. Similarly, conven-tional nuclear medicine modalities possess subopti-mal spatial resolution in assessing the viability of small grafts. [18F]-fluoride PET is proven to be able to monitor the viability of osseous structures [68,69]. For this reason, dynamic fluoride PET has been used with great success for the evaluation of bone allograft viability and metabolism [70,71]. It has been shown that fluoride PET is a sensitive method for the evaluation of bone formation in allogenic bone grafts early after hip revision arthro-plasty [70,71]. In addition, [15O]-water PET can be used in the evaluation of bone blood flow to the allograft in such a clinical setting [71].

Summary

PET is an important imaging modality for assessing the success of arthroplasty. The discrepancy in the results reported by different groups is mainly caused by the specific variation in the diagnostic criteria used by these investigators. As optimal standards for diagnosing periprosthetic infection are adopted by the imaging community, FDG-PET should play a crucial role in distinguishing aseptic loosening from periprosthetic infection. In addition, PET might be useful in the evaluation of bone graft after revision arthroplasty.

References

[1] Andrews HJ, Arden GP, Hart GM, et al. Deep infection after total hip replacement. J Bone Joint Surg Br 1981;63:53–7.

[2] Maderazo EG, Judson S, Pasternak H. Late infections of total joint prostheses. A review and recommendation for prevention. Clin Orthop 1988;229:131–42.

[3] Brown SR, Davies WA, DeHeer DH, et al. Long-term survival of McKee-Farrar total hip prostheses. Clin Orthop 2002;402:157–63.

[4] Mahomed NN, Barrett JA, Katz JN, et al. Rates and outcomes of primary and revision total hip replacement in the United States Medicare population. J Bone Joint Surg Am 2003;85:27–32.

[5] Furnes O, Lie SA, Espehaug B, et al. Hip disease and the prognosis of total hip replacements. A review of 53,698 primary total hip replacements reported to the Norwegian Arthroplasty Register 1987–99. J Bone Joint Surg Br 2001;83:579–86.

[6] Fehring TK, Cohen B. Aspiration as a guide to sepsis in revision total hip arthroplasty. J Arthroplasty 1996;11:543–7.

[7] Spangehl MJ, Younger ASE, Masri BA, et al. Diagnosis of infection following total hip arthroplasty. J Bone Joint Surg Am 1997;79:1587–8.

[8] Barrack RL, Jennings RW, Wolfe MW, et al. The value of preoperative aspiration before total knee revision. Clin Orthop 1997;345:8–16.

[9] Kraemer WJ, Saplys R, Waddell JP, et al. Bone scan, gallium scan, and hip aspiration in the diagnosis of infected total hip arthroplasty. J Arthroplasty 1993;8:611–6.

[10] Reinartz P, Mumme T, Hermanns B, et al. Radionuclide imaging of the painful hip arthroplasty. J Bone Joint Surg Br 2005;87:465–70.

[11] Palestro CJ, Roumanas P, Swyer AJ, et al. Diagnosis of musculoskeletal infection using combined In-111 labeled leukocyte and Tc-99m SC marrow imaging. Clin Nucl Med 1992;17:269–73.

[12] Mulamba LAH, Ferrant A, Lencers N, et al. Indium-111-leukocyte scanning in the evaluation of painful hip arthroplasty. Acta Orthop Scand 1983;54:695–7.

[13] Achong DM, Oates E. The computer-generated bone marrow subtraction image: a valuable adjunct to combined in-111 WBC/Tc-99m in sulfur colloid scintigraphy for musculoskeletal infection. Clin Nucl Med 1994;19:188–93.

[14] Palestro CJ, Kim CK, Swyer AJ, et al. Total-hip arthroplasty: periprosthetic indium-111 labeled leukocyte activity and complementary technetium-99m-sulfur colloid imaging in suspected infection. J Nucl Med 1990;31:1950–4.

[15] Alazraki NP. Diagnosing prosthetic joint infection. J Nucl Med 1990;31:1955–7.

[16] Bakheet SM, Saleem M, Powe J, et al. F-18 fluorodeoxyglucose chest uptake in lung inflammation and infection. Clin Nucl Med 2000;25:273–8.

[17] Zhuang H, Cunnane ME, Ghesani NV, et al. Chest tube insertion as a potential source of false-positive FDG-positron emission tomographic results. Clin Nucl Med 2002;27:285–6.

[18] Dadparvar S, Anderson GS, Bhargava P, et al. Paraneoplastic encephalitis associated with cystic teratoma is detected by fluorodeoxyglucose positron emission tomography with negative magnetic resonance image findings. Clin Nucl Med 2003;28:893–6.

[19] Yu JQ, Kumar R, Xiu Y, et al. Diffuse FDG uptake in the lungs in aspiration pneumonia on positron emission tomographic imaging. Clin Nucl Med 2004;29:567–8.

[20] Bleeker-Rovers CP, de Kleijn E, Corstens FHM, et al. Clinical value of FDG PET in patients with fever of unknown origin and patients suspected of focal infection or inflammation. Eur J Nucl Med Mol Imaging 2004;31:29–37.

[21] Tsai YF, Wu CC, Su CT, et al. FDG PET CT features of an intraabdominal gossypiboma. Clin Nucl Med 2005;30:561–3.

[22] Nguyen QH, Szeto E, Mansberg R, et al. Paravertebral infection (phlegmon) demonstrated by FDG dual-head coincidence imaging in a patient with multiple malignancies. Clin Nucl Med 2005;30:241–3.

[23] Yu JQ, Kung JW, Potenta S, et al. Chronic cholecystitis detected by FDG-PET. Clin Nucl Med 2004;29:496–7.

[24] Zhuang H, Alavi A. 18-Fluorodeoxyglucose positron emission tomographic imaging in the detection and monitoring of infection and inflammation. Semin Nucl Med 2002;32:47–59.

[25] Zhuang H, Yu JQ, Alavi A. Applications of fluorodeoxyglucose-PET imaging in the detection of infection and inflammation and other benign disorders. Radiol Clin North Am 2005;43:121–34.

[26] De Winter F, Gemmel F, Van De Wiele C, et al. 18-Fluorine fluorodeoxyglucose positron emission tomography for the diagnosis of infection in the postoperative spine. Spine 2003;28:1314–9.

[27] Meller J, Koster G, Liersch T, et al. Chronic bacterial osteomyelitis: prospective comparison of F-18-FDG imaging with a dual-head coincidence camera and In-111-labelled autologous leucocyte scintigraphy. Eur J Nucl Med 2002;29:53–60.

[28] Guhlmann A, Brecht-Krauss D, Suger G, et al. Fluorine-18-FDG PET and technetium-99m antigranulocyte antibody scintigraphy in chronic osteomyelitis. J Nucl Med 1998;39:2145–52.

[29] Kalicke T, Schmitz A, Risse JH, et al. Fluorine-18 fluorodeoxyglucose PET in infectious bone diseases: results of histologically confirmed cases. Eur J Nucl Med 2000;27:524–8.

[30] Temmerman OPP, Heyligers IC, Hoekstra OS, et al. Detection of osteomyelitis using (18)FDG and positron emission tomography. J Arthroplasty 2001;16:243–6.

[31] Zhuang H, Duarte PS, Pourdehand M, et al. Exclusion of chronic osteomyelitis with F-18 fluorodeoxyglucose positron emission tomographic imaging. Clin Nucl Med 2000;25:281–4.

[32] Gratz S, Dorner J, Fischer U, et al. F-18-FDG hybrid PET in patients with suspected spondylitis. Eur J Nucl Med Mol Imaging 2002;29:516–24.

[33] Keidar Z, Militianu D, Melamed E, et al. The diabetic foot: initial experience with F-18-FDG PET/CT. J Nucl Med 2005;46:444–9.

[34] Koort JK, Makinen TJ, Knuuti J, et al. Comparative F-18-FDG PET of experimental Staphylococcus aureus osteomyelitis and normal bone healing. J Nucl Med 2004;45:1406–11.

[35] Jones-Jackson L, Walker R, Purnell G, et al. Early detection of bone infection and differentiation from post-surgical inflammation using 2-deoxy-2-[(18)F]-fluoro-D-glucose positron emission tomography (FDG-PET) in an animal model. J Orthop Res 2005;23(6):1484–9.

[36] Sahlmann CO, Siefker U, Lehmann K, et al. Dual time point 2-F-18 fluoro-2′-deoxyglucose positron emission tomography in chronic bacterial osteomyelitis. Nucl Med Commun 2004;25:819–23.

[37] Xiu Y, Yu JQ, Cheng E, et al. Sarcoidosis demonstrated by FDG PET imaging with negative findings on gallium scintigraphy. Clin Nucl Med 2005;30:193–5.

[38] Chacho TK, Zhuang H, Nakhoda KZ, et al. Application of fluorodeoxyglucose positron emission tomography in the diagnosis of infection. Nucl Med Commun 2003;24:615–24.

[39] Chacko TK, Zhuang HM, Alavi A. FDG-PET is an effective alternative to WBC imaging in diagnosing and excluding orthopedic infections. [abstract]. J Nucl Med 2002;43:458.

[40] Schiesser M, Stumpe KDM, Trentz O, et al. Detection of metallic implant-associated infections with FDG PET in patients with trauma: correlation with microbiologic results. Radiology 2003;226:391–8.

[41] Zhuang H, Duarte PS, Pourdehnad M, et al. The promising role of F-18-FDG PET in detecting infected lower limb prosthesis implants. J Nucl Med 2001;42:44–8.

[42] Reddy S, Hochhold J, Pill S, et al. The value of FDG-PET imaging in the evaluation of infection associated with hip arthroplasty. J Nucl Med 2005;46:324P.

[43] Vanquickenborne B, Maes A, Nuyts J, et al. The value of (18)FDG-PET for the detection of infected hip prosthesis. Eur J Nucl Med Mol Imaging 2003;30:705–15.

[44] Stumpe K, Nötzli H, Zanetti M, et al. FDG PET for differentiation of infection and aseptic loosening in total hip replacements: comparison with conventional radiography and three-phase bone scintigraphy. Radiology 2004;231:333–41.

[45] Zhuang H, Chacko TK, Hickeson M, et al. Persistent non-specific FDG uptake on PET imaging following hip arthroplasty. Eur J Nucl Med Mol Imaging 2002;29:1328–33.

[46] Revell PA, Weightman B, Freeman MA, et al. The production and biology of polyethylene wear debris. Arch Orthop Trauma Surg 1978; 91:167–81.

[47] Kisielinski K, Cremerius U, Reinartz P, et al. Fluorodeoxyglucose positron emission tomography detection of inflammatory reactions due to polyethylene wear in total hip arthroplasty. J Arthroplasty 2003;18:528–32.

[48] Kisielinski K, Reinartz P, Mumme T, et al. The FDG-PET demonstrates foreign body reactions to particulate polyethylene debris in uninfected knee prostheses. Nuklearmedizin 2004;43: N3–6.

[49] Chacko TK, Zhuang H, Stevenson K, et al. The importance of the location of fluorodeoxyglucose uptake in periprosthetic infection in painful hip prostheses. Nucl Med Commun 2002;23:851–5.

[50] Mumme T, Reinartz P, Alfer J, et al. Diagnostic values of positron emission tomography versus triple-phase bone scan in hip arthroplasty loosening. Arch Orthop Trauma Surg 2005;125:322–9.

[51] Chacko TK, Zhuang H, Nakhoda KZ, et al. Applications of fluorodeoxyglucose positron emission tomography in the diagnosis of infection. Nucl Med Commun 2003;24:615–24.

[52] De Winter F, Van de Wiele C, De Clercq D, et al. Aseptic loosening of a knee prosthesis as imaged on FDG positron emission tomography. Clin Nucl Med 2000;25:923.

[53] Van Acker F, Nuyts J, Maes A, et al. FDG-PET, 99mtc-HMPAO white blood cell SPET and bone scintigraphy in the evaluation of painful total knee arthroplasties. Eur J Nucl Med 2001; 28:1496–504.

[54] Heiba SI, Luo JQ, Sadek S, et al. Attenuation correction induced artifact in F-18 FDG PET imaging following total knee replacement. Clin Positron Imaging 2000;3:237–9.

[55] Manthey N, Reinhard P, Moog F, et al. The use of F-18 fluorodeoxyglucose positron emission tomography to differentiate between synovitis, loosening and infection of hip and knee prostheses. Nucl Med Commun 2002;23:645–53.

[56] Love C, Marwin SE, Tomas MB, et al. Diagnosing infection in the failed joint replacement: a comparison of coincidence detection F-18-FDG and In-111-labeled leukocyte/Tc-99m-sulfur colloid marrow imaging. J Nucl Med 2004;45:1864–71.

[57] Goerres GW, Schmid DT, Eyrich GK. Do hardware artefacts influence the performance of head and neck PET scans in patients with oral cavity squamous cell cancer? Dentomaxillofac Radiol 2003;32:365–71.

[58] Bockisch A, Beyer T, Antoch G, et al. Positron emission tomography/computed tomography-imaging protocols, artifacts, and pitfalls. Mol Imaging Biol 2004;6:188–99.

[59] Kamel EM, Burger C, Buck A, et al. Impact of metallic dental implants on CT-based attenuation correction in a combined PET/CT scanner. Eur Radiol 2003;13:724–8.

[60] Halpern BS, Dahlbom M, Waldherr C, et al. Cardiac pacemakers and central venous lines can induce focal artifacts on CT-corrected PET images. J Nucl Med 2004;45:290–3.

[61] Rubash HE, Sinha RK, Shanbhag AS, et al. Pathogenesis of bone loss after total hip arthroplasty. Orthop Clin North Am 1998;29: 173–86.

[62] Gamradt SC, Lieberman JR. Bone graft for revision hip arthroplasty: biology and future applications. Clin Orthop 2003;417:183–94.

[63] Toms AD, Barker RL, Jones RS, et al. Impaction bone-grafting in revision joint replacement surgery. J Bone Joint Surg Am 2004;86: 2050–60.

[64] Schreurs BW, Arts JJ, Verdonschot N, et al. Femoral component revision with use of impaction bone-grafting and a cemented polished stem. J Bone Joint Surg Am 2005;87:2499–507.

[65] Leopold SS, Jacobs JJ, Rosenberg AG. Cancellous allograft in revision total hip arthroplasty. A clinical review. Clin Orthop 2000;371:86–97.

[66] Heekin RD, Engh CA, Vinh T. Morselized allograft in acetabular reconstruction. A postmortem retrieval analysis. Clin Orthop 1995;319:184–90.

[67] Hooten JP Jr, Engh CA, Heekin RD, et al. Structural bulk allografts in acetabular reconstruction. Analysis of two grafts retrieved at post-mortem. J Bone Joint Surg Br 1996;78:270–5.

[68] Schliephake H, Berding G, Knapp WH, et al. Monitoring of graft perfusion and osteoblast activity in revascularised fibula segments using [18F]-positron emission tomography. Int J Oral Maxillofac Surg 1999;28:349–55.

[69] Hawkins RA, Choi Y, Huang SC, et al. Evaluation of the skeletal kinetics of fluorine-18-fluoride ion with PET. J Nucl Med 1992;33:633–42.

[70] Piert M, Winter E, Becker GA, et al. Allogenic bone graft viability after hip revision arthroplasty assessed by dynamic [18F]fluoride ion positron emission tomography. Eur J Nucl Med 1999;26:615–24.

[71] Sorensen J, Ullmark G, Langstrom B, et al. Rapid bone and blood flow formation in impacted morselized allografts: positron emission tomography (PET) studies on allografts in 5 femoral component revisions of total hip arthroplasty. Acta Orthop Scand 2003;74:633–64.

RADIOLOGIC
CLINICS
OF NORTH AMERICA

Radiol Clin N Am 45 (2007) 719–733

Nonprosthesis Orthopedic Applications of ^{18}F Fluoro-2-Deoxy-D-Glucose PET in the Detection of Osteomyelitis

Johannes Meller, MD[a],*, Carsten Oliver Sahlmann, MD[a],
Torsten Liersch, MD[b], Peter Hao Tang, BA[c], Abass Alavi, MD[c]

- Clinical background
  Bacterial osteomyelitis
- Pathophysiologic basis of
  [^{18}F]2-fluoro-2-deoxy-D-glucose uptake in infection and inflammation
  *Metabolic basis for
  [^{18}F]2-fluoro-2-deoxy-D-glucose uptake*
  Biodistribution
  Uptake of [^{18}F]2-fluoro-2-deoxy-D-glucose in inflammatory cells
  Influence of serum glucose levels and insulin

- *Summary*
- Uptake of [^{18}F]2-fluoro-2-deoxy-D-glucose during fracture healing and after bone surgery
  Physiology of bone healing
  Preclinical studies
  Clinical studies
- Clinical studies in osteomyelitis
  Acute osteomyelitis
  Chronic osteomyelitis
  Chronic recurrent multifocal osteomyelitis
- Summary
- References

Imaging for the diagnosis of orthopedic inflammation and infection dates back to the 1970s when modern imaging techniques were introduced. To this day, a three-phase bone scan is commonly used in the evaluation of OM of the intact bone. With the advent of white blood cell (WBC) labeling techniques, a relatively specific modality for orthopedic infection became available in the late 1970s. The complexities of labeling WBCs, poor spatial resolution, and the difficulties in differentiating between soft tissue and bone involvement are major limitations of this method.

It has long been recognized that FDG accumulates not only in malignant tissues but at the sites of inflammation and infection, but systematic assessment of this method in diagnosing infection has only been undertaken over the past decade. This review describes the impact of FDG-PET in the diagnosis of non–prosthesis-related orthopedic infection as reported in the literature.

This article was previously published in PET Clinics 2006;1:107–22.
[a] Department of Nuclear Medicine, University of Göttingen, Robert Koch-Straße 40, D- 37075, Göttingen, Germany
[b] Department of General Surgery, University of Göttingen, Göttingen, Germany
[c] Division of Nuclear Medicine, Department of Radiology, Hospital of the University of Pennsylvania, 110 Donner Building, 3400 Spruce Street, Philadelphia, PA 19104, USA
* Corresponding author.
E-mail address: jmeller@med.uni-goettingen.de (J. Meller).

doi:10.1016/j.rcl.2007.05.011

Clinical background

Bacterial osteomyelitis

OM is an acute or chronic inflammatory process of the bone marrow and adjacent bone attributable to pyogenic organisms. It is usually classified into several types based on the patient's age, onset of disease, route of infection, and etiology.

Known predisposing factors for OM are diabetes mellitus, AIDS, intravenous drug abuse, alcoholism, chronic steroid use, immunosuppression, chronic joint disease, any recent orthopedic surgery or open fractures, and the presence of prosthetic orthopedic devices [1,2].

Dependent on the route of inoculation and infections agents, OM is divided into hematogenous (endogenous) and nonhematogenous (exogenous) types. Hematogenous OM of an intact bone is seen most often in the extremities in neonates and children and in the spine of immunocompromised patients (spondylodiscitis). Nonhematogenous OM, which is appropriately better termed *ostitis* because the bone marrow is only infrequently involved, is the consequence of contiguous spread of infection from the adjacent soft tissue infection.

Bacterial types found in hematogenous OM include *Staphylococcus aureus*, *Streptococcus* variants, *Haemophilus influenzae*, and *Enterobacter* species. Exogenous OM (ostitis) is more often caused by *S aureus*, *Enterobacter* species, and *Pseudomonas* species [1–5].

Based on the appropriate clinical settings, the onset of symptoms, and the degree of inflammation, the process is described as acute, subacute, or chronic [1–4]. The distinction between acute OM and chronic osteomyelitis (COM) is somewhat arbitrary. Some patients with an acute clinical course show histologic findings suggestive of chronic disease, and during exacerbation of COM, focal polymorphonuclear infiltration would suggest acute infection [3].

Acute hematogenous osteomyelitis

Hematogenous OM is an infection caused by bacterial seeding from the blood. This occurs primarily in children and in the intact bone. The most common site of infection is the metaphysis of the long bones, which is highly vascular. The process begins with the implantation of microorganisms and a neutrophilic response. This is accompanied by local edema, vasospasm, and thrombosis. Segmental ischemic necrosis or sequestrum may follow soon after the process starts. The infection may be localized, or it may spread through the periosteum, cortex, marrow, and cancellous tissue. Depending on the child's age and the blood supply to the epiphysis, the process may or may not affect the adjacent joint. In children between the ages of 1 and approximately 16 years, the blood supply to the metaphysis and epiphysis is separate; therefore, spread of the microorganisms to the adjacent joint is rare. Conversely, in infants less than 1 year of age and in adults, there is a common blood supply to the metaphysis and epiphysis, and no growth plate barrier exists in this population. The presence of this communication facilitates the spread of infection to adjacent joints [1–6].

Acute exogenous osteomyelitis (ostitis)

The bone is highly resistant to infection, which can only occur as a result of direct contact between bone tissue and bacteria during trauma or surgery. Bacteria like *S aureus* adhere to the damaged bone by expressing various binding components, such as collagen, fibrinonectin, and others. Once the microorganisms adhere to the bone, they express phenotypic resistance to antimicrobial drugs, which may partly explain the high failure rate of antibiotic therapy of such infections [6].

Bone invasion by microorganisms is facilitated by focal osteolysis, which is caused by activated osteoclasts that are stimulated by cytokines released from the inflammatory cells. The disintegration of the surrounding bone matrix caused by proteolytic enzymes secreted by phagocytes further propagates bacterial invasion. Secondarily, the process may affect the bone marrow and lead to bone marrow phlegmon and other complications similar to those described for hematogenous OM. Clinical manifestations of ostitis are often localized compared with hematogenous OM, and multiple organisms are often noted at the site [1,2,4,5].

Chronic osteomyelitis

There is no generally accepted definition for COM, which is an expression that best describes bone and marrow infections and is based on histologic, clinical, and etiologic parameters [2,4,5]. COM is frequently the result of inadequate treatment of acute hematogenous OM or may follow exogenous bacterial contamination caused by trauma or surgical procedures. In contrast to acute OM, COM is predominantly characterized by the presence of lymphocytic and plasmacellular infiltrates and a variable amount of necrosis and osteosclerosis. In chronic recurrent cases, neutrophil infiltration may also be present. The presence of necrotic tissue may lead to draining fistulas or to organization in the medullary cavity, forming Brodie's abscesses [1,2,5]. Although, clinically, there is a frequent overlap between acute and chronic inflammatory changes, COM can be assumed if evidence of infection is present for more than 2 to 6 weeks. [1,3,5,7].

Vertebral osteomyelitis

Spondylodiscitis is an infection of the intervertebral disk and the adjacent vertebral bodies. The most commonly affected site is the lumbar spine. The disease occurs more frequently in older patients, especially in those who are immunocompromised. Most cases are caused by hematogenous bacterial spread from a distant site; however, in recent years, such infections have been noted after back surgery. The clinical course is usually rather subacute; therefore, the diagnosis is often delayed. The microorganisms are introduced by the arterial rather than the venous routes, and early infection is usually located in the subchondral zone of the end plate of the vertebral body, an area that is richly supplied with nutrient end arteries. The infection usually rapidly spreads to the adjacent vertebra above or below the disk space. Pyogenic spondylodiscitis virtually always involves two adjacent segments of the spine [3].

Chronic osteomyelitis and the diabetic foot

Approximately 15% of diabetics develop foot OM, which most commonly involves the metatarsal bones and proximal phalanges. In addition to impaired leukocyte function in these patients, OM is often the consequence of a condition called the "diabetic foot." Diabetic foot is a complex bone and joint disorder that involves the foot and ankle in patients with long-standing diabetes caused by neuropathy that affects the peripheral sensory, motor, and autonomic nerves. Eventually, this disorder leads to repetitive unnoticed damage and trauma without protective reflexes, imbalances in the arch of the foot with altered weight distribution and foot pressures, and deficient sweat production that causes thick and dry skin and callus formation in areas of pressure. Neuropathy combined with impaired arterial circulation and repetitive trauma is the major contributor to skin fissures and ulcer formation. More than 90% of OM of the foot in diabetics occurs as a result of infected ulcers, which lead to subsequent COM of the adjacent bone [6].

Pathophysiologic basis of [^{18}F]2-fluoro-2-deoxy-D-glucose uptake in infection and inflammation

Metabolic basis for [^{18}F]2-fluoro-2-deoxy-D-glucose uptake

FDG is structurally an analogue of glucose; therefore, it is taken up according to the degree of glycogen in the body.

The uptake of glucose and FDG into mammalian cells takes place via three mechanisms of transport. The first, passive diffusion, is of minor importance for human tissues. The second, active transport by a Na$^+$-dependent glucose transporter, is of importance in the kidney epithelial cells and intestinal tract. The third and most significant pathway for FDG to enter human cells is active transport mediated by facilitated glucose transporters (GLUT-1–10) [8].

Once FDG has entered the cell, it is subsequently phosphorylated to 2′-FDG-6 phosphate by the hexokinase enzyme. In contrast to glucose-6-phosphate, 2′-FDG-6 phosphate is not a substrate for the enzymes of the glycolytic pathway or the pentose-phosphate shunt. In tissues with low concentrations of the glucose-6-phosphatase enzyme, such as the heart and brain, the uptake of 2′-FDG-6 phosphate increases over time. In other organs with high concentrations of the enzyme, such as the liver, the uptake of 2′-FDG-6 phosphate decreases after the rapid initial accumulation [9,10].

Biodistribution

FDG is filtrated in the glomeruli in the kidneys, and only a small fraction is reabsorbed by the renal tubular cells. Rapid clearance of the tracer from the vascular compartment results in a high target-to-background ratio within a short time; therefore, imaging can start as early as 30 to 60 minutes after injection.

A high accumulation of FDG is always seen in the brain, especially in the gray matter. Cardiac uptake is unpredictable in patients who have fasted before dose administration. If the patient exercises before the administration of the tracer, muscular uptake may be high. Because of renal excretion, the kidney, pelvis, and urinary bladder are usually visualized on FDG scans. Variable levels of FDG uptake are seen in the gastrointestinal tract, which may interfere with correct interpretation of the scan, is likely attributable to smooth muscle peristalsis, and can be reduced by the administration of N-butylscopolamine [11].

Tracer uptake in the reticuloendothelial system (RES), and especially in the red bone marrow, is significant. In patients with fever, bone marrow uptake is usually high, probably as a consequence of interleukin-dependent upregulation of glucose transporters [Fig. 1] [12]. The cortical bone and cavity of the long tubular bones are usually free of activity [Fig. 2]. Systematic studies on the uptake in the normal synovia of healthy individuals have not been reported in literature. It has been recognized, however that a faint FDG uptake is almost always present in the synovial portion of the joints. The uptake may be related to normal glucose consumption in the tissue, but osteoarthritis should be considered as the basis for this observation [13].

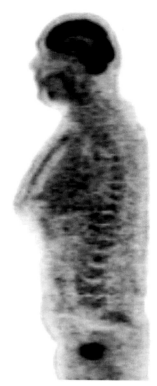

Fig. 1. In patients with normal hematopoietic activity, there is usually a low degree of uptake in the axial bone marrow. If the bone marrow is activated by cytokines, as in this patient with fever of unknown origin, the uptake may be high, which may result in false-negative findings. In this patient with OM, FDG uptake in the lesions was obscured because of increased background activity within the third and fourth vertebral bodies of the lumbar spine (PET sagittal view).

Uptake of [¹⁸F]2-fluoro-2-deoxy-D-glucose in inflammatory cells

It has long been recognized that FDG accumulates not only in malignant tissues but at the sites of inflammation and infection [14,15]. A few studies have made an attempt to clarify the mechanism of FDG uptake in the inflammatory cells in vitro [16–18]. In these experiments, mixed preparations of WBCs or pure preparations of neutrophils and mononuclear cells were used for this purpose. In these research studies, the labeling efficiency ranged from 40% to 80% [16–18]. If a mixed population of nonstimulated WBCs is incubated with FDG, labeling is predominantly attributable to granulocytic uptake, accounting for 78% to 87% of the activity in the preparation. The labeling efficiency depends on the amount of activity in the media and the experimental temperature, with the maximum labeling efficiency achievable at 37°C. The

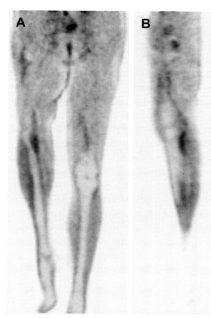

Fig. 2. Normal pattern in the peripheral bone on FDG-PET. The long bones are usually free of any activity. The uptake near the cortical bone in the maximal projection image (A) is clearly related to vascular activity, as demonstrated on the sagittal view (B).

uptake increases within the first 60 minutes [16, 18]. The extent of uptake by neutrophilic granulocytes is inversely proportional to the glucose concentration in the labeling medium [16]. Insulin, even in high concentrations, does not increase the uptake in the inflammatory cells [17].

If neutrophilic granulocytes are stimulated by substances like phorbol myristate or the chemotactic peptide N-formyl-methionyl-leucyl-phenylalanine (f-MLP) for a relatively short period of 60 minutes, a significant increase in FDG uptake is noted compared with nonstimulated cells [16,18].

The labeling of WBCs with FDG is not stable, and an elution of 27% to 35% within the first 60 minutes has been reported [16,18]. Osman and Danpure [16] demonstrated that after the initial intracellular uptake and phosphorylation of FDG in WBCs, it is then dephosphorylated by the glucose-6-phosphatase and leaves the cells again. Because of this poor stability, cells labeled with FDG in vitro are not suited for clinical application, although some authors have advocated their use for clinical purposes [17]. The functionality of the labeled cells after reinjection is another open question.

Currently, autoradiographic data about differential uptake of FDG in inflammatory cell elements are limited. In a microautoradiographic study,

Kubota and colleagues [19] demonstrated that the tracer uptake in tumors was partly attributable to newly formed granulation tissue and activated macrophages associated with tumor necrosis and growth. In this study, the FDG uptake of nonneo-plastic cell elements was even higher than the accumulation of the tracer in viable tumor cells. In another report, FDG uptake in postmigratory and activated leukocytes in lobar pneumonia was autoradiographically shown to be localized within neutrophils [20].

Activated lymphocytes in concanavalin A–medi-ated acute inflammatory tissues showed increased uptake of FDG in in vitro and in vivo models [21]. In an animal model of bacterial infection induced by inoculation with *Escherichia coli*, auto-radiographs showed that the highest [^{3}H]-FDG uptake was in the area of inflammatory cell infiltra-tion surrounding the necrotic region [22].

In recent years, many aspects of the molecular basis of FDG uptake in WBCs have been successfully clarified. As already discussed, the transport of glucose and structurally related substances like FDG into mammalian cells is mediated by faculta-tive glucose transporters (GLUT-1–10) [8]. GLUT-1 is the most common isotype and is thought to play a major role in the basal glucose supply of many fetal and adult tissues. The expression of GLUT-1 has been especially demonstrated in the brain, the cells of the blood-brain barrier, and the blood, par-ticularly in erythrocytes but also in the leukocyte fraction [23].

GLUT-1 seems to be the target of many cytokines and the most important isotype for our understanding of FDG uptake in WBCs, especially after stimulation. Overexpression of GLUT-1 after stimulation with cytokines or mutagens has already been demonstrated in vitro in murine and human macrophages [24–26] as well as in human lympho-cytes and neutrophils [27,28].

GLUT-1 is located predominantly in the plasma membrane but can also be found within intracellu-lar vesicles [26]. After stimulation, the intracellular GLUT-1 pool can be translocated to the cell mem-brane, thus increasing glucose transport capacity within a relatively short time [12]. If human lym-phocytes are stimulated with mitogens, this effect takes place as early as 30 minutes after the begin-ning of stimulation [29]. This may explain the early increase of FDG uptake in cultured WBCs in vitro.

In addition to these early stimulatory effects, the late (>24 hours) increase in FDG uptake in stimu-lated inflammatory cells in vitro is attributable to a gene-dependent de novo synthesis of GLUT-1. This has already been demonstrated on an mRNA and protein level for lymphocytes [27], where the maximal overexpression of GLUT-1 was observed

for murine and human monocytes as late as 48 hours after stimulation [24–26]. Similar results were found in neutrophilic granulocytes and cellu-lar elements of granulation tissue, such as fibro-blasts and the endothelium [30–33].

In human tuberculosis lesions, the GLUT-1– positive staining was often localized in the mem-branes of neutrophils and macrophages around necrotizing granulomas as well as in the cytoplasm. These cells also showed positive staining for the hexokinase II (HK-II) isoform, which is known to play a dominant role in the accelerated phosphory-lation of FDG in tumor cells [28].

GLUT-3 has a high affinity for glucose and can be found in a wide range of tissues, especially in the kidney, the placenta, and the neurons in the brain, where it ensures a constant glucose supply even at low extracellular glucose concentrations [17].

In a monocyte-macrophage cell line, GLUT-3 affinity for glucose was found to be enhanced during the respiratory burst [34], whereas nonsti-mulated WBCs usually did not express this type of transporter [27].

Mochizuki and coworkers [35] used a suspension of *S aureus* in rats to induce soft tissue infection. Other animals were inoculated with allogenic hep-atoma cells into the left calf muscle. The expression of glucose transporters (GLUT-1–5) was investi-gated by immunostaining the infectious and tumor tissues. In this study, the [^{14}C]FDG uptake was sig-nificantly higher in the tumor than in the inflam-matory lesion. The tumor and inflammatory tissues highly expressed GLUT-1 and GLUT-3. The GLUT-1 expression level was, however, significantly higher in the tumor tissue than in the inflammatory tissue. The GLUT-3 levels tended to be higher in the inflammatory lesions than in the tumor, but the difference did not reach statistical significance.

Influence of serum glucose levels and insulin

High serum glucose levels decrease glucose uptake in experimental inflammatory and infectious lesi-ons because of decreased GLUT-1 (inflammatory lesions of noninfectious origin) and GLUT-3 (in-flammatory lesions of infectious origin) expression [36]. Whether or not this observation is of clinical importance remains an open question. Based on their in vitro and in vivo data, Zhuang and co-workers [37] concluded that contrary to observa-tions in malignant disorders, below a level of 250 mg/dL, elevated glucose concentration does not have a negative effect on FDG uptake in inflamma-tory cells.

Hyperinsulinemia increases the level of glucose uptake in GLUT-4–rich organs like the heart, fat, and muscles by translocation of GLUT-4 from intra-cellular vesicles to the membrane and therefore

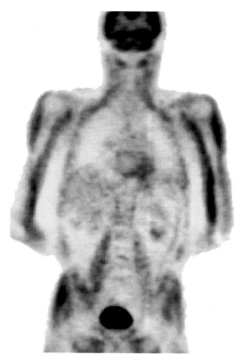

Fig. 3. FDG-PET images (coronal view) of a 72-year-old patient with spondylodiscitis in the lumbar spine. A false-negative result in this affected site is attributable to hyperinsulinemia. Maximal FDG uptake is found in the skeletal muscles by upregulation of the GLUT-4 isotype.

shifts the uptake from inflammatory lesions toward these tissues [36]. This mechanism leads to false-negative results in FDG-PET imaging [Fig. 3].

Summary

In summary, migratory and postmigratory inflammatory cells stimulated by cytokines show an overexpression of GLUT-1 and GLUT-3 and an activation of the glycolytic pathway. These mechanisms of enhanced FDG uptake are of essential importance in PET imaging of acute and chronic bacterial infection. Although the expression of glucose transporters is insulin sensitive to a certain degree, in vivo data indicate that serum glucose levels below a certain level may not adversely affect the image quality for inflammatory lesions.

Uptake of [^{18}F]2-fluoro-2-deoxy-D-glucose during fracture healing and after bone surgery

Physiology of bone healing

Fracture healing is a complex process that involves the coordinated participation of several cell types. It begins with an inflammatory phase, followed by repair and remodeling, and culminates in the ability of bone to regain its original tissue structure. Fracture healing begins immediately after injury when interleukins and growth factors are released into the fracture hematoma by platelets and inflammatory cells. Growth factors are regulators of cellular proliferation, differentiation, and extracellular matrix synthesis during fracture repair. The most important of these are the bone morphogenetic proteins (BMPs), transforming growth factor-β (TGFβ), platelet-derived growth factor (PDGF), fibroblast growth factor (FGF), insulin-like growth factor (IGF), vascular endothelial growth factor (VEGF), and epidermal growth factor (EGF). Altered growth factor expression may be responsible for abnormal or delayed fracture repair. Intramembranous ossification occurs under the periosteum within a few days after an injury. Endochondral ossification occurs adjacent to the fracture site and spans a period of up to 1 month [38].

Preclinical studies

Systematic preclinical studies on FDG uptake in the healing bone after fracture and surgery are infrequently reported in the literature.

Jones-Jackson and coworkers [39] used a rabbit OM model and a dual–time-point FDG-PET protocol to differentiate between postsurgical inflammation and infection of the bone. Comparisons were made between noninfected and infected rabbits in which infection with S aureus was initiated at the time of surgery. Increased uptake of FDG was evident in the bone of all rabbits on day 1 after surgery; however, the standardized uptake value (SUV) could not be used to distinguish between the infected and uninfected groups until day 15.

Koort and colleagues [40] compared the natural course of bone healing after creating a metaphyseal defect in the tibia of rabbits without (control group) and after the inoculation of S aureus (OM group). Before surgery, the SUVs of FDG did not differ markedly between the right and left tibias. In the controls, uncomplicated bone healing was associated with a temporary increase in FDG uptake in the third week, with almost complete normalization by week 6. In the OM group, localized infection resulted in an intense continuous uptake of FDG, which was significantly higher than that of the healing and intact bones at weeks 3 and 6.

Clinical studies

The first clinical data on FDG uptake in the traumatized bone are concordant with those of the experimental observations [41–50]. Fig. 4 shows a false-positive finding in a patient with a history of fracture less than 3 weeks old [see Fig. 4].

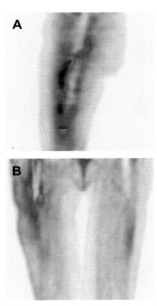

Fig. 4. FDG-PET in a 38-year-old patient with a recent fracture of the right femur and soft tissue infection of the surrounding soft tissue (*A*, sagittal view; *B*, coronal view). Although soft tissue infection was proven by surgery, the uptake in the bone was posttraumatic and not related to infection.

In a series of 29 patients with known fractures, no false-positive findings were noted in 5 patients who underwent bone surgery within 3 to 28 weeks before FDG-PET with a coincidence camera [44].

In a study by Zhuang and coworkers [48] in 22 patients with fractures, 2 with a recent osteotomy showed false-positive FDG uptake, whereas a negative scan ruled out infection in the remaining 20 subjects.

In another report in 60 patients with suspected OM, FDG-PET allowed correct identification of OM in 25 patients, but 2 of 3 patients with false-positive findings had undergone bone surgery less than 6 weeks and 4 months before PET imaging [42].

In a prospective series of 16 patients with suspected spondylitis who underwent FDG-PET with a coincidence camera, one false-positive finding was noted and was attributed to a vertebral fracture of unknown age [47].

In another prospective FDG-PET study of 57 patients with a history of previous spinal surgery, false-positive findings occurred in 2 of 27 patients without metallic implants within the first 6 months after surgery. A negative PET scan had a negative predictive value of 100% [43].

In a retrospective study in 37 patients with known fractures, the pattern and time course of abnormal FDG uptake after traumatic or surgical

fracture were assessed. Fourteen patients had fractures or surgery within 3 months before FDG-PET, whereas 23 had fractures or surgical intervention more than 3 months before FDG-PET. FDG-PET showed normal uptake at the known fracture or surgical site(s) in 30 patients. In the 23 patients with fractures more than 3 months old, all but 1 showed no abnormally increased uptake. This patient had a complicated case of OM. Six of the 14 patients with a history of fracture less than 3 months old had abnormally increased FDG uptake despite normal fracture healing [49].

Schmitz and colleagues [50] evaluated FDG-PET findings in patients with osteoporosis and acute (<3 weeks) vertebral compression fractures. The results of blind scoring of FDG uptake at the fracture sites were compared with those of MRI, which served as the "gold standard." In 13 of 17 patients, MRI demonstrated an osteoporotic fracture. Twelve of 13 PET scans in these patients were scored as 0 or 1 (no uptake or uptake slightly increased) and were categorized as true-negative findings in patients with uncomplicated fractures. The maximum SUV ranged from 1.1 to 2.4. In the remaining 4 patients, MRI revealed a pathologic fracture caused by spondylodiscitis in 3 patients and by plasmocytoma in 1 patient. In these patients, FDG-PET scans were highly positive and the maximum SUV values ranged from 3.8 to 9.8.

In summary, less than 50% of patients with uncomplicated traumatic or surgical fractures demonstrate pathologic FDG uptake within the first 3 months after bone injury. During this time, interval reparative changes of the bone are usually characterized by low FDG uptake and by maximum SUV values less than 2. Intense uptake and higher maximum SUV values at a fracture site for longer than 3 months are suspicious for infection or other pathologic processes, such as malignancy. Our present knowledge about possible differences in the time course of enhanced FDG uptake after trauma to the bone in different sites is limited. The glucose metabolism of the axial and peripheral skeleton after trauma may be different. Another open question is how different mechanical forces at different sites may affect glucose metabolism of the healing bone. In a study on postoperative fever, we noted distinct FDG uptake after an uncomplicated sternotomy in 3 patients up to 5 weeks after surgery, which could have been easily confused with the presence of OM [45].

Clinical studies in osteomyelitis

Acute osteomyelitis

Acute OM, especially that of the intact bone, can readily be diagnosed by the combination of physical examination, laboratory findings, and three-phase bone scanning or MRI. The role of FDG-PET in acute infection of the bone is limited, because conventional imaging techniques have a diagnostic accuracy of more than 90% [15,46].

In a study describing 15 patients with histopathologically proven OM, 7 had acute infection of the spine or the perpendicular skeleton. All cases in this highly selected patient population were detected by FDG-PET [51]. Except for these seven cases, publications about FDG-PET in acute OM have been limited to the animal models already described [39,40]. Without data of larger prospective studies, it is impossible to define a possible role for FDG-PET in the diagnosis of acute bone and marrow infection.

Chronic osteomyelitis

Using conventional imaging methods, including MRI and labeled leukocyte scanning, the diagnosis of COM remains a diagnostic challenge.

In the context of COM, bone scintigraphy is sensitive, and a negative bone scan can rule out infection in almost all cases. Conversely, a low specificity of 18% to 62% has been reported for the bone scan in the diagnosis of COM [46,52,53]. In vitro radiolabeled leukocytes or immunoscintigraphy with in vivo labeling antigranulocyte antibodies has proven to be accurate in the diagnosis of COM in the peripheral skeleton but lacks sensitivity and specificity in the axial bones [6,15].

The sites of chronic infection in the axial skeleton are usually characterized by an area of decreased activity on the WBC scan. This pattern is nondiagnostic for active inflammation because it may also be found in other conditions, such as healing OM, fibrosis, fatty bone marrow degeneration, metastases, primary tumors of the bone, and osteonecrosis [6,46]. Decreased uptake of labeled cells in infection of the axial skeletal compartment is poorly understood. This is likely attributable to relatively high uptake of FDG in the red marrow compared with the site of infection. Other explanations include microthrombotic occlusion and inflammatory compression of the blood capillaries, which prevent the migration of labeled cells or antibodies to the site of infection [6,15,46]. Conversely, FDG uptake in active OM is usually enhanced, whereas glycolysis in the surrounding bone marrow is relatively low, which allows for the detection of lesions that are missed in WBC imaging [Figs. 5 and 6].

MRI has been recognized as an extremely sensitive modality for the detection of COM; compared with nuclear medicine techniques, it provides more accurate anatomic information about the extent of the process and possible complications [52,53]. The criteria used to identify inflammatory

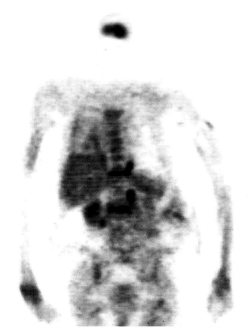

Fig. 5. FDG-PET images (coronal view) of a 62-year-old patient with multifocal OM of the spine and soft tissue involvement of the adjacent areas.

changes, such as the edema pattern on T2-weighted sequences and contrast enhancement after intravenous administration of gadolinium, are unspecific, however, and may produce false-positive results, especially in the first year after surgery.

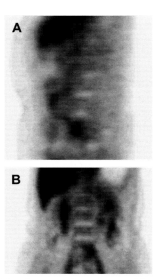

Fig. 6. FDG-PET images of a 48-year-old patient with OM of the ventral lumbosacral junction extending to the soft tissue. (*A*, sagittal view; *B*, coronal view).

Furthermore, artifacts produced by metallic implants hinder correct interpretation [52,53].

Guhlmann and coworkers [54] were the first to publish a prospective study about the possible role of FDG-PET in the diagnosis of COM. They evaluated the results of FDG-PET and antigranulocyte antibody scintigraphy in 51 patients. COM was suspected if OM was recurrent or if symptoms lasted for more than 6 weeks. Patients who had undergone bone surgery within the past 2 years were excluded. In 31 patients, histologic findings or the results of bacterial culture were available. For image interpretation, a visual score was used. The findings were evaluated by two independent readers who were blinded to the final diagnosis. Excellent accuracy and interobserver agreement for both techniques (97% and 95% for FDG-PET and 86% and 92% for antigranulocyte antibody scintigraphy, respectively) were noted in the peripheral skeleton (n = 36). In the axial skeleton (n = 15), accuracy was significantly higher for FDG-PET (93% and 100%) than for antigranulocyte antibody scintigraphy (73% and 80%; P<.05).

In another publication by the same group, in 31 patients suspected of having COM in the peripheral (n = 21) or axial (n = 10) skeleton and having available histology results, the overall sensitivity and specificity of FDG-PET were 100% and 92%, respectively. The one false-positive case was in a patient with a soft tissue infection of the mandible. This was explained by a lack of the missing landmarks of FDG-PET in this region [55]. Again, patients with previous bone surgery within the past 12 months before PET imaging were excluded, which may explain the low rate of false-positive findings in this and the previous study.

Zhuang and colleagues [48] investigated 22 patients with possible COM (axial skeleton [n = 11] or peripheral skeleton [n = 11]). The final diagnosis was made by surgical exploration or clinical follow-up during a 1-year period. FDG-PET correctly diagnosed all 6 patients with COM. There were two false-positive findings, resulting in a sensitivity, specificity, and accuracy of 100%, 87.5%, and 91%, respectively. The two false-positive findings were caused by a recent osteotomy.

Kälicke and coworkers [51] reported the results of FDG-PET in 15 histologically confirmed cases of infection (8 with COM and 7 with acute OM). The authors provided no definition of acute and OM. The PET findings were evaluated by two independent readers, blinded to the results of other imaging modalities. Image interpretation was performed by using a semiquantitative score. FDG-PET yielded true-positive results in all 15 patients. The absence of negative findings in this series may raise questions concerning selection criteria, however.

De Winter and coworkers [41] prospectively evaluated the role of the dual-headed coincidence (DHC) imaging system versus the role of a dedicated PET device in 24 patients with suspected chronic orthopedic infection. A final diagnosis in this study was obtained by microbiologic proof in 11 patients and clinical follow-up in 13 patients. The sensitivity and specificity in this series were 100% and 86% for the dedicated PET and 89% and 96% for the DHC, respectively. These results indicate that DHC imaging, despite a lower imaging quality, can be used successfully in the evaluation of orthopedic infections in most cases.

The same group published a prospective study of 60 patients in whom COM, spondylodiscitis, or infection of a total joint prosthesis was suspected [42]. Microbiologic and histopathologic findings were available for 42 patients. In 24 patients, detailed clinical follow-up confirmed the diagnosis. Suspected COM was defined as a possible recurrence of previously known disease or the presence of typical symptoms for more than 6 weeks. Patients with recent bone surgery were not excluded. FDG images were evaluated visually by two independent readers blinded to the final diagnosis. Twenty-five patients had infection, and 35 did not. All 25 infections were correctly identified by both readers. There were four false-positive findings; in two of these cases, surgery had been performed less than 6 months before the study. The sensitivity and specificity for the 33 patients with a suspected infection of the axial skeleton were 100% and 90%, respectively. The sensitivity and specificity for the 13 patients with a suspected infection of the peripheral skeleton were 100% and 86%, respectively.

Schmitz and colleagues [56] performed FDG-PET in 16 patients with suspected spondylodiscitis. Surgery and histopathologic examination were performed in all patients. The FDG-PET findings were semiquantitatively graded and evaluated by two independent readers. Of the 16 patients, 12 had histopathologically confirmed spondylodiscitis. There were true-positive FDG-PET findings in all 12 of these patients. In the 4 patients without spondylodiscitis, FDG-PET showed three true-negative results and one false-positive result.

Meller and coworkers [44] published a prospective analysis of 29 consecutive nondiabetic patients who were studied for possible COM and underwent combined indium (In)-111 WBC imaging and FDG-PET with a DHC imaging system. In 4 patients, bone surgery had been performed within the past 6 months. All patients complained of localized symptoms for more than 6 weeks. Image interpretation was performed semiquantitatively by two investigators who were blinded to the results of other diagnostic modalities and the final diagnosis.

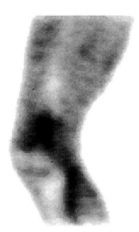

Fig. 7. FDG coincidence imaging with a DHC imaging system (sagittal slices) 30 minutes after injection of FDG (sagittal slices) in a 44-year-old patient with COM in the distal femur.

Of 34 regions with suspected infection, 13 were localized in the axial skeleton and 21 in the peripheral skeleton [Figs. 7 and 8]. COM was proven in 10 of 34 regions and subsequently excluded in 24 of 34 regions. The final diagnosis was established by histologic examination and culture in 18 regions and by MRI and clinical follow-up in 16 regions. The sensitivity of PET imaging was 100%, and the specificity was 95%. Results of ^{111}In WBC imaging were inferior, especially in the axial skeleton.

In a prospective study of 17 patients with histopathologically proven COM of the axial skeleton, our group used a dual-time protocol to evaluate the tracer kinetics of FDG in chronic bacterial OM compared with the kinetics of bone metastases [Figs. 9–11]. In all infectious lesions, increased FDG uptake was seen at 30 and 90 minutes after the injection of FDG. In COM lesions, the maximum SUV and mean SUV between 30 and 90 minutes after injection remained stable or decreased in 16 of 17 patients. Changes in the maximum SUV and mean SUV between 30 and 90 minutes were

highly significant ($P<.05$). In 1 patient, the maximum SUV and mean SUV increased over the time. The histologic examination of this patient revealed multiple foreign body granulomas in addition to a mononuclear infiltrate. In malignant lesions, the maximum SUV and mean SUV between 30 and 90 minutes after injection increased. From these limited results, we concluded that a dual-time protocol should allow differentiation between infectious and malignant lesions of the spine in most cases [57].

The great potential of FDG-PET in postoperative patients can be derived from the data provided by de Winter and colleagues [43] in 57 consecutive patients with a history of previous spinal surgery who underwent FDG-PET in the postoperative period. Of these patients, 15 had a spinal infection, whereas infection could be ruled out in the others. Images were semiquantitatively and visually scored by two blinded independent readers. Using the most sensitive cutoff values, sensitivity, specificity, and accuracy were 100%, 81%, and 86%, respectively, for visual and semiquantitative scoring.

Direct comparisons between FDG-PET and MRI are of great importance, because PET may overcome some of the limitations of MRI as described previously.

One patient who developed COM and ostitis after repeated osteosynthesis in a fibular transplant underwent MRI, antigranulocyte antibody scintigraphy, and FDG PET. Infection of the fibular transplant was demonstrated by PET but not by the other methods [58].

Our group prospectively studied 12 patients with suspected COM. FDG-PET was as sensitive as but more specific than MRI (100% versus 60%) [44]. In a retrospective study of 14 patients after surgery of the spine, the sensitivity of FDG-PET and MRI was 87%, whereas the specificity of PET was superior to that of MRI (100% versus 85%) [59]. Larger prospective studies in a population of patients that should include cases after bone surgery are therefore clearly warranted.

A 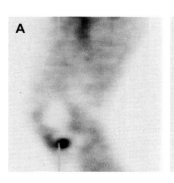 **B**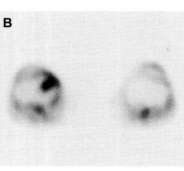

Fig. 8. FDG coincidence imaging with a DHC imaging system (sagittal slices) 120 minutes after injection of FDG in a 35-year-old patient with COM in the right proximal tibia (*A*, sagittal view; *B*, transversal view).

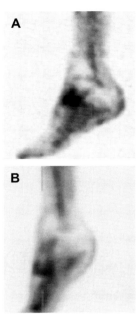

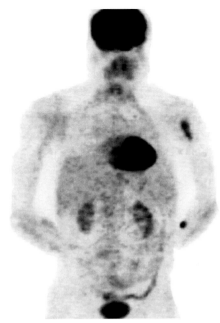

Fig. 9. FDG-PET (dual-time protocol 30 minutes and 60 minutes after injection, sagittal slices) in a 63-year-old patient with tarsal COM. The extent of the inflammatory uptake and the SUV decreased with time (*A*, 30 minutes after injection, maximum SUV = 4.22; *B*, 90 minutes after injection, maximum SUV = 3.58).

Fig. 11. FDG-PET images of a patient with COM in the proximal left humerus 90 minutes after injection of FDG (coronal view).

Chronic recurrent multifocal osteomyelitis

Chronic recurrent multifocal osteomyelitis (CRMO) has been described as a self-limited relapsing inflammatory condition histologically characterized by a mononuclear cell infiltrate and usually affecting children and adolescents [6]. A nonbacterial origin for CRMO is probable but not proven. Most of the lesions are seen in the long bones, especially in the tibia. The clavicle is often bilaterally involved. Fig. 12 shows one of the three patients who underwent combined bone scintigraphy, antigranulocyte antibody scintigraphy, and FDG-PET in our institution. Although the bone scan was positive in all known lesions, the antigranulocyte antibody scintigraphy showed decreased uptake at the sites of inflammation. FDG-PET was completely negative in all lesions, indicating low metabolic activation of the lymphoplasmacellular infiltrate [see Fig. 12].

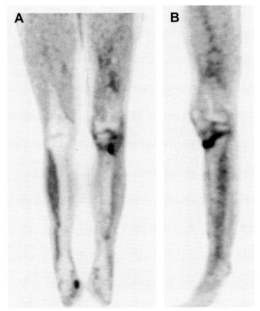

Fig. 10. FDG-PET images of a 67-year-old patient with COM in the proximal tibia 90 minutes after injection of FDG (*A*, coronal view; *B*, sagittal view). Note the presence of osteoarthritis of the right hallux.

Summary

FDG-PET imaging seems to have excellent sensitivity in the detection of COM. A normal scan virtually rules out infection. FDG-PET is superior to scintigraphy with labeled blood cells in the diagnosis of COM in the axial skeleton and should thus be considered the method of choice for this indication. This seems to hold true for peripheral lesions as well, but the number of cases published to date is

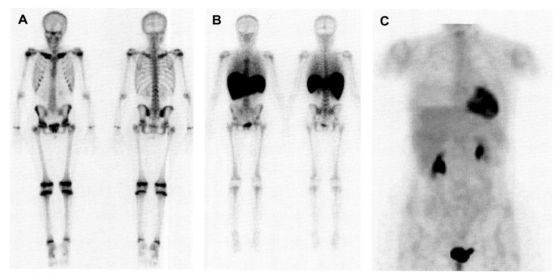

Fig. 12. CRMO in both clavicles in an 18-year-old male patient. The bone scan (*A*) was positive in the clavicular lesions, and the antigranulocyte antibody scintigraphy (*B*) showed decreased uptake at the sites of inflammation. (*C*) Maximal projection FDG-PET image was completely negative.

too small to permit a final conclusion. FDG-PET is likely to become the standard technique in the diagnosis of COM in the near future.

Compared with labeled blood cells, FDG-PET has some important advantages:

- Diagnosis can be performed within a short period (1–2 hours after injection).
- From a theoretic point of view, it can be assumed that labeled WBCs only accumulate in COM if sufficient blood flow is present at the site of infection and if the chemotactic-guided emigration of labeled cells from the blood pool to the inflammatory tissue is still ongoing. FDG, as a small molecule, is expected to be much more independent of microcirculatory changes and can label activated postmigratory granulocytes and mononuclear cells in the inflammatory tissue sites.
- Compared with conventional gamma camera imaging, PET offers higher spatial and contrast resolutions. As a rule, no FDG uptake can be observed in the normal bone and uptake in the axial bone marrow is low. The target-to-background ratio in infectious lesions on the FDG scan is thus higher than that of the labeled images.
- When labeled cells are used to delineate infectious processes in the axial skeleton, the diseased sites appear to be negative compared with the surrounding background because of uptake of WBCs in the hematopoietic bone marrow. This pattern results in low sensitivity for the labeled cell technique.

Conversely, active OM in the axial skeleton can be clearly visualized by FDG-PET in almost all cases because of substantially increased glucose metabolism at the sites of infection compared with the normal bone marrow.

- Uptake of labeled WBCs in the hematopoietic bone marrow in the peripheral skeleton poses a problem when using labeled leukocytes. Low-grade infection in these areas may be missed because of unfavorable target-to-background ratios with this technique. FDG shows minimal uptake in the bone marrow of the peripheral skeleton; therefore, such confusion can be avoided.
- Low-grade infection or infection with purely mononuclear or granulomatous infiltrates may be missed on WBC scanning. It is well known that FDG uptake is generally preserved in these conditions and is independent of chemotactic stimuli.

Traumatic or surgical fracture has been found to be the most frequent cause of false-positive findings on FDG-PET in the context of evaluation for COM. Careful interpretation of the scan using semiquantitative or quantitative methods may avoid false-positive results in many cases, but differentiating between infection and inflammation is an issue that may not be feasible with PET, especially in the first 4 to 6 weeks after trauma.

Early data indicate that FDG-PET may be more specific than MRI in diagnosing COM. In general, MRI can only show tissue edema and hyperperfusion and is thus not specific in this context. FDG-PET is taken up in postmigratory inflammatory cells, and the uptake in the tissue is independent of such phenomena. This allows a unique opportunity to detect the primarily elements at the site of infection. Larger prospective studies are clearly warranted to clarify this matter.

The significance of low-uptake lesions on FDG-PET with a normal appearance on MRI has not been fully elucidated, because these are usually categorized as false-positive findings and may not require further investigation. It may well be possible that lesions with low FDG uptake represent ongoing infection and are related to exacerbation of a latent disease.

The use of PET-CT in the assessment of infections processes should further enhance the role of the technique for this indication. In particular, this methodology should be of great importance in separating soft tissue infection from that of the musculoskeletal structures.

References

[1] Lew DP, Waldvogel FA. Osteomyelitis. N Engl J Med 1997;336(14):999–1007.

[2] Lew DP, Waldvogel FA. Osteomyelitis. Lancet 2004;364(9431):369–79.

[3] Waldvogel FA, Medoff G, Swartz MN. Osteomyelitis: a review of clinical features, therapeutic considerations and unusual aspects. N Engl J Med 1970;282(4):316–22.

[4] Waldvogel FA, Vasey H. Osteomyelitis: the past decade. N Engl J Med 1980;303(7):360–71.

[5] Mader JT, Shirtliff M, Calhoun JH. Staging and staging application in osteomyelitis. Clin Infect Dis 1997;25(6):1303–9.

[6] Becker W. Imaging osteomyelitis and the diabetic foot. Q J Nucl Med 1999;43(1):9–20.

[7] Schauwecker DS. The scintigraphic diagnosis of osteomyelitis. AJR Am J Roentgenol 1992;158(1):9–18.

[8] Shepherd PR, Kahn BB. Glucose transporters and insulin action: implications for insulin resistance and diabetes mellitus. N Engl J Med 1999;341(4):248–57.

[9] Sokoloff L, Reivich M, Kennedy C, et al. The (14C) deoxyglucose method for the measurement of local cerebral glucose utilisation: theory, procedure and normal values in the conscious and anesthetized albino rat. J Neurochem 1977;28(6):897–916.

[10] Pauwels EK, Sturm EJ, Bombardieri E, et al. Positron-emission tomography with fluorodeoxyglucose. Part I. Biochemical uptake mechanism and its implication for clinical studies. J Cancer Res Clin Oncol 2000;126(10):549–59.

[11] Stahl A, Weber WA, Avril N, et al. Effect of N-butylscopolamine on intestinal uptake of fluorine-18-fluorodeoxyglucose in PET imaging of the abdomen. Nuklearmedizin 2000;39(8):241–5.

[12] Baldwin SA, Kan O, Whetton AD, et al. Regulation of the glucose transporter GUT1 in mammalian cells. Biochem Soc Trans 1994;22(3):814–7.

[13] von Schulthess GK, Stumpe KDM, Engel-Bicik I. Clinical PET imaging of inflammatory diseases. In: von Schulthess GK, editor. Clinical positron emission tomography (PET). Philadelphia: Lippincott Williams & Wilkins; 2000. p. 229–48.

[14] Tahara T, Ichiya Y, Kuwabara Y, et al. High-fluorodeoxyglucose uptake in abdominal abscesses: a PET study. J Comput Assist Tomogr 1989;13(5):829–31.

[15] Becker W, Meller J. The role of nuclear medicine in infection and inflammation. Lancet Infect Dis 2001;1(1):326–33.

[16] Osman S, Danpure HJ. The use of 2-fluoro-2-deoxy-D-glucose as a potential in vitro agent for labelling human granulocytes for clinical studies by positron emission tomography. Int J Radiat Appl Instrum 1992;19(2 Pt B):183–90.

[17] Forstrom LA, Mullan BP, Hung JC, et al. ^{18}F-FDG labelling of human leucocytes. Nucl Med Commun 2000;21(7):691–4.

[18] Lehmann K, Meller J, Behe M, et al. F-18-FDG uptake in granulozyten: basis der F-18-FDG szintigraphie. Nuklearmedizin 2001;40(3):V168 [in German].

[19] Kubota R, Yamada S, Kubota K, et al. Intratumoral distribution of fluorine-18-fluorodeoxyglucose in vivo: high accumulation in macrophages and granulocytes studied by microautoradiography. J Nucl Med 1992;33(7):1972–80.

[20] Jones HA, Sriskandan S, Peters AM, et al. Dissociation of neutrophil emigration and metabolic activity in lobar pneumonia and bronchiectasis. Eur Respir J 1997;10(4):795–803.

[21] Ishimori T, Saga T, Mamede M, et al. Increased (18)F-FDG uptake in a model of inflammation: concanavalin A-mediated lymphocyte activation. J Nucl Med 2002;43(5):658–63.

[22] Sugawara Y, Gutowski TD, Fisher SJ, et al. Uptake of positron emission tomography tracers in experimental bacterial infections: a comparative biodistribution study of radiolabeled FDG, thymidine, L-methionine, 67Ga-citrate, and 125I-HSA. Eur J Nucl Med 1999;26(4):333–41.

[23] Gould GW, Holman GD. The glucose transporter family: structure, function and tissue-specific expression. Biochem J 1993;295:329–41.

[24] Gamelli RL, Liu H, He LK, et al. Augmentations of glucose uptake and glucose transporter-1 in macrophages following thermal injury and sepsis in mice. J Leukoc Biol 1996;59(5):639–47.

[25] Fukuzumi M, Shinomiya H, Shimizu Y, et al. Endotoxin-induced enhancement of glucose influx into murine peritoneal macrophages via GLUT1. Infect Immun 1996;64(1):108–12.

[26] Malide D, Davies-Hill TM, Levine M, et al. Distinct localisation of GLUT-1 and -5 in human

monocyte-derived macrophages: effects of cell activation. Am J Physiol 1998;274(3 Pt 1):E516–26.

[27] Chakrabarti R, Jung CY, Lee TP, et al. Changes in glucose transport and transporter isoforms during the activation of human peripheral blood lymphocytes by phytohemagglutinin. J Immunol 1994;152(6):2660–8.

[28] Mamede M, Higashi T, Kitaichi M, et al. FDG uptake and PCNA, Glut-1, and Hexokinase-II expressions in cancers and inflammatory lesions of the lung. Neoplasia 2005;7(4):369–79.

[29] Jacobs DB, Lee TP, Jung CY, et al. Mechanism of mitogen-induced stimulation of glucose transport in human peripheral blood mononuclear cells. J Clin Invest 1989;83(2):437–43.

[30] Pekala P, Marlow M, Heuvelman D, et al. Regulation of hexose transport in aortic endothelial cells by vascular permeability factor and tumor necrosis factor-alpha, but not by insulin. J Biol Chem 1990;265(30):18051–4.

[31] Cornelius P, Marlowe M, Pekala PH. Regulation of glucose transport by tumor necrosis factor-α in cultured murine 3T3–L1 fibroblasts. J Trauma 1990;30(12 Suppl):S15–20.

[32] Tan AS, Ahmed N, Berridge MV. Acute regulation of glucose transport after activation of human peripheral blood neutrophils by phorbol myristate acetate, fMLP, and granulocyte-macrophage colony-stimulating factor. Blood 1998;91(2):649–55.

[33] Bird TA, Davies A, Baldwin SA, et al. Interleukin 1 stimulates hexose transport in fibroblasts by increasing the expression of glucose transporters. J Biol Chem 1990;265(23):13578–83.

[34] Ahmed N, Kansara M, Berridge MV. Acute regulation of glucose transport in a monocyte-macrophage cell line: Glut-3 affinity for glucose is enhanced during the respiratory burst. Biochem J 1997;327:369–75.

[35] Mochizuki T, Tsukamoto E, Kuge Y, et al. FDG uptake and glucose transporter subtype expressions in experimental tumor and inflammation models. J Nucl Med 2001;42(10):1551–5.

[36] Zhao S, Kuge Y, Tsukamoto E, et al. Fluorodeoxyglucose uptake and glucose transporter expression in experimental inflammatory lesions and malignant tumours: effects of insulin and glucose loading. Nucl Med Commun 2002;23(6):545–50.

[37] Zhuang HM, Cortes-Blanco A, Pourdehnad M, et al. Do high glucose levels have differential effect on FDG uptake in inflammatory and malignant disorders? Nucl Med Commun 2001;22(10):1123–8.

[38] Einhorn TA. The cell and molecular biology of fracture healing. Clin Orthop 1998;355(Suppl):S7–21.

[39] Jones-Jackson L, Walker R, Purnell G, et al. Early detection of bone infection and differentiation from post-surgical inflammation using 2-deoxy-2-[(18)F]-fluoro-d-glucose positron emission tomography (FDG PET) in an animal model. J Orthop Res 2005;23(6):1484–9.

[40] Koort JK, Makinen TJ, Knuuti J, et al. Comparative 18F-FDG PET of experimental Staphylococcus aureus osteomyelitis and normal bone healing. J Nucl Med 2004;45(8):1406–11.

[41] de Winter F, Van de Wiele C, Vandenberghe S, et al. Coincidence camera FDG imaging for the diagnosis of chronic orthopedic infections: a feasibility study. J Comput Assist Tomogr 2001;25(2):184–9.

[42] de Winter F, van de Wiele C, Vogelaers D, et al. Fluorine-18 fluorodeoxyglucose-position emission tomography: a highly accurate imaging modality for the diagnosis of chronic musculoskeletal infections. J Bone Joint Surg Am 2001;83(5):651–60.

[43] de Winter F, Gemme F, Van De Wiele C, et al. 18-Fluorine fluorodeoxyglucose positron emission tomography for the diagnosis of infection in the postoperative spine. Spine 2003;28(12):1314–9.

[44] Meller J, Köster G, Liersch T, et al. Chronic bacterial osteomyelitis—prospective comparison of 18 FDG-imaging with a double head coincidence camera (DHCC) and In-111 labeled autologous leucocytes. Eur J Nucl Med 2002;29(1):53–60.

[45] Meller J, Sahlmann CO, Lehmann K, et al. F-18-FDG hybrid camera PET in patients with postoperative fever. Nuklearmedizin 2001;41(1):22–9.

[46] Meller J, Siefker U, Becker W. Nuklearmedizinische Diagnostik erregerbedingter Skeletterkrankungen [Scientific diagnosis of bacterial skeletal diseases]. Nuklearmedizin 2002;25(2):122–32 [in German].

[47] Gratz S, Dörner J, Fischer U, et al. 18F-FDG hybrid PET in patients with suspected spondylitis. Eur J Nucl Med 2002;29(4):516–24.

[48] Zhuang H, Duarte PS, Pourdehand M, et al. Exclusion of chronic osteomyelitis with F-18 fluorodeoxyglucose positron emission tomographic imaging. Clin Nucl Med 2000;25(4):281–4.

[49] Zhuang H, Sam JW, Chacko TK, et al. Rapid normalization of osseous FDG uptake following traumatic or surgical fractures. Eur J Nucl Med Mol Imaging 2003;30(8):1096–103.

[50] Schmitz A, Risse JH, Textor J, et al. FDG PET findings of vertebral compression fractures in osteoporosis: preliminary results. Osteoporos Int 2002;13(9):755–61.

[51] Kälicke T, Schmitz A, Risse JH, et al. Fluorine-18 fluorodeoxyglucose PET in infectious bone diseases: results of histologically confirmed cases. Eur J Nucl Med 2000;27(5):524–8.

[52] Kaim A, Ledermann HP, Bongartz G, et al. Chronic post-traumatic osteomyelitis of the lower extremity: comparison of magnetic resonance imaging and combined bone scintigraphy/immunoscintigraphy with radiolabelled monoclonal antigranulocyte antibodies. Skeletal Radiol 2000;29(7):378–86.

[53] Kaim AH, Gross T, von Schulthess GK. Imaging of chronic posttraumatic osteomyelitis. Eur Radiol 2003;13(7):1750–2.

[54] Guhlmann A, Brecht Krauss D, Suger G, et al. Fluorine-18-FDG PET and technetium-99m antigranulocyte antibody scintigraphy in chronic osteomyelitis. J Nucl Med 1998;39(12): 2145–52.

[55] Guhlmann A, Brecht-Krauss D, Suger G, et al. Chronic osteomyelitis: detection with FDG PET and correlation with histopathologic findings. Radiology 1998;206(3):749–54.

[56] Schmitz A, Risse JH, Grunwald F, et al. Fluorine-18 fluorodeoxyglucose positron emission tomography findings in spondylodiscitis: preliminary results. Eur Spine J 2001;10(6):534–9.

[57] Sahlmann CO, Siefker U, Lehmann K, et al. Dual time point 2-[^{18}F]fluoro-2′-deoxyglucose ([^{18}F] FDG)-PET in chronic bacterial osteomyelitis (COM). Nucl Med Commun 2004;25(8):819–23.

[58] Robiller FC, Stumpe KD, Kossmann T, et al. Chronic osteomyelitis of the femur: value of PET imaging. Eur Radiol 2000;10(5):855–8.

[59] Siefker U, Sahlmann CO, Lehmann K, et al. F-18-FDG PET im Vergleich zur MRT bei der Primärdiagnostik und postoperativen Kontrolle bei chronischer bakterieller Osteomyelitis (COM). Nuklearmedizin 2004;43(3):V116 [in German].

RADIOLOGIC CLINICS OF NORTH AMERICA

Radiol Clin N Am 45 (2007) 735–744

[¹⁸F]Fluorodeoxyglucose PET in Large Vessel Vasculitis

Martin A. Walter, MD

- Giant cell arteritis
- Takayasu's arteritis
- Diagnostic workup in large vessel vasculitis
- [¹⁸F]fluorodeoxyglucose PET
- [¹⁸F]fluorodeoxyglucose PET scanning protocols for large vessel vasculitis
- [¹⁸F]fluorodeoxyglucose PET and atherosclerosis

- [¹⁸F]fluorodeoxyglucose PET for diagnosing giant cell arteritis
- [¹⁸F]fluorodeoxyglucose PET for diagnosing Takayasu's arteritis
- [¹⁸F]fluorodeoxyglucose PET CT in large vessel vasculitis
- Summary
- Acknowledgments
- References

[¹⁸F]fluorodeoxyglucose (FDG) PET is a noninvasive metabolic imaging modality based on the regional distribution of [¹⁸F]FDG and has become increasingly important in the management of oncologic patients [1]. Remarkable images of patients with active vasculitis have been generated through [¹⁸F]FDG-PET scans [2–10]. These images indicate the potential of this technique and imply that [¹⁸F]FDG-PET may soon be useful in evaluating patients with several forms of vasculitis, especially large vessel vasculitis.

The family of vasculitides has been defined with reference to the size of vessels involved in large, medium, and small vessel vasculitis [Table 1]. The group of large vessel vasculitides includes giant cell arteritis and Takayasu's arteritis. Both of these diseases are challenging with respect to their diagnosis and follow-up, because affected patients regularly present with a set of nonspecific symptoms and laboratory test results. Consequently, a delayed or even unsuccessful diagnostic workup occurs in several patients. The use of whole-body scanning via [¹⁸F]FDG-PET might facilitate a sensitive metabolic imaging modality that could lead to a shorter and more successful diagnostic workup in the near future.

The current data on [¹⁸F]FDG-PET in large vessel vasculitis are still sparse, however. The results of only 12 clinical trials are currently available [Table 2]. In addition, there are no standardized guidelines existing for the indication, performance, interpretation, and description of [¹⁸F]FDG-PET in large vessel vasculitis. Therefore, the purpose of this review is to summarize current information on the present clinical data and to assist nuclear medicine and rheumatology practitioners in recommending, performing, and interpreting the results of [¹⁸F]FDG-PET in patients with suspected large vessel vasculitis.

Giant cell arteritis

Giant cell arteritis is a granulomatous vasculitis of large- and medium-sized arteries that was first described by Hutchinson [11] in 1890. It usually affects the cranial branches of the arteries originating from the aortic arch, particularly the superficial temporal artery; nevertheless, involvement of the entire aorta and its main branches occurs in

This article was previously published in PET Clinics 2006;1:179–90.
Institute of Nuclear Medicine, University Hospital, Petersgraben 4, Basel CH-4031, Switzerland
E-mail address: m.a.walter@gmx.net

doi:10.1016/j.rcl.2007.05.012

Table 1: Classification of vasculitis

Size of vessels	Type of vasculitis	Classification criteria[a]
Large	Giant cell arteritis	Age at onset of disease ≥50 years New headache Temporal artery abnormality Elevated erythrocyte sedimentation rate Abnormal findings on biopsy of temporal artery
	Takayasu's arteritis	Age at onset of disease ≤40 years Claudication of an extremity Decreased brachial artery pulse Difference in systolic blood pressure between arms Bruit over the subclavian arteries or the aorta Narrowing or occlusion of the entire aorta at angiography
Medium	Periarteritis nodosa Kawasaki's arteritis Primary central nervous system vasculitis Buerger's disease	
Small	Wegener's disease Churg-Strauss syndrome Microscopic polyangiitis Henoch-Schönlein purpura Essential cryoglobulinemic vasculitis Cutaneous leukocytoclastic angiitis	

[a] Diagnosis of giant cell arteritis: at least three of five criteria: sensitivity of 93.5%, specificity of 90.5%. Diagnosis of Takayasu's arteritis: at least three of six criteria: sensitivity of 91.2%, specificity of 97.8%.

approximately 15% of cases [12]. Giant cell arteritis commonly occurs in the white population, with an incidence of approximately 18 per 100,000 persons in the population aged older than 50 years [13-15]; however, autopsy studies suggest that it may be more common than is clinically apparent [16]. It rarely occurs in Asians and blacks, and women are affected twice as often as men [13]. Until now, the etiology of giant cell arteritis has remained unknown. The classic histologic picture is granulomatous inflammation in which giant cells are usually located at the connection between the intima and

Table 2: Clinical studies on PET in the detection of large vessel inflammation: the present literature

Authors	Year	Takayasu's arteritis	Giant cell arteritis	Follow-up scans	Reference
Blockmans et al	1999	—	11[a]	—	[62]
Blockmans et al	2000	—	25[a]	—	[63]
Belhocine et al	2002	—	3	3	[64]
Meller et al	2003	5	—	—	[51]
Meller et al	2003	1	14	7	[47]
Bleeker-Rovers et al	2003	1	7[a]	1	[44]
Webb et al	2004	18	—	8	[43]
Brodman et al	2004	—	22	—	[45]
Moosig et al	2004	—	12[a]	8	[46]
Andrews et al	2004	6	—	6	[42]
Scheel et al	2004	—	8	8	[52]
Kobayashi et al	2005	14	—	7	[49]
Walter et al	2005	6	20	4	[48]
Blockmans et al	2006	—	35[a]	22	[65]
Total		51	122	52	

[a] Patients with giant cell arteritis and polymyalgia rheumatica.

media. Panarteritides with mixed-cell inflammatory infiltrates of lymphomononuclear cells, with occasional neutrophils and eosinophils but without giant cells, are also found [17]. The focal arteritic lesions cause ischemia and subsequently lead to a variety of systemic manifestations, whereas the onset of symptoms may be sudden or gradual. Systemic symptoms are present in most patients [18,19]; among these, headache is probably the most frequent symptom and occurs in two thirds of patients [19]. The symptoms also include myalgia, neck pain, scalp tenderness, jaw claudication, fever, abnormal temporal arteries, polyneuropathy of the arms and legs, transient ischemic attacks, general malaise, fatigue, anorexia, weight loss, depression, and night sweats [18,20,21].

Takayasu's arteritis

Takayasu's arteritis is a large vessel vasculitis that primarily affects the aorta and its main branches as well as the coronary and pulmonary arteries. It is named for Mikito Takayasu, who reported the peculiar wreath-like arteriovenous anastomoses around the papillae in a young woman with pulseless disease in 1908 [22]. The incidence of the disease is approximately 2 per 1,000,000 population, with a mean age at onset of 35 years [23–25] and a prevalence in women approximately 10 times higher than in men. Takayasu's arteritis has a worldwide distribution, although it is considered to be more common in the Orient [26]. Its etiology remains unresolved, and its clinical course includes an early and late phase. Pathology studies in the early phase reveal granulomatous or diffuse productive inflammation in the media and adventitia, with secondary thickening of the intima and occasional perivascular inflammation [27]. Commonly, clinical findings include fever of unknown origin with nonspecific systemic symptoms. Conversely, pathology studies in the late phase show marked thinning of the media, with disruption of elastic fibers, fibrotic thickening of the adventitia, and marked intimal proliferation [27]. Variable ischemic symptoms secondary to arterial stenosis or occlusion or arterial dilatation and aneurysmal formation cause various clinical morbid conditions, such as arm claudication, decreased artery pulses, carotodynia, visual loss, stroke, aortic regurgitation, and hypertension [28]. The topologic classification of Takayasu's arteritis is based on angiographic findings [29], with involvement of branches of the aortic arch (type I); the ascending aorta and the aortic arch and its branches (type IIa); the ascending aorta, the aortic arch and its branches, and the thoracic descending aorta (type IIb); the thoracic descending aorta, the abdominal aorta, or renal arteries (type III); the abdominal aorta or renal arteries (type IV); or combined features of types IIb and IV.

Diagnostic workup in large vessel vasculitis

Giant cell arteritis and Takayasu's arteritis usually present with a wide clinical spectrum; except for the histopathologic findings, there are no laboratory findings specific for either disease. A set of clinical, radiologic, and histologic criteria has been established by the American College of Rheumatology to classify cases of biopsy-proven arteritis [see Table 1] [30,31]. The presence of at least three criteria is required for classifying a patient as having Takayasu's arteritis or giant cell arteritis. These criteria provide a sensitivity of 93.5% with a specificity of 90.5% for diagnosing giant cell arteritis and a sensitivity of 91.2% with a specificity of 97.8% for diagnosing Takayasu's arteritis in biopsy-positive patients. Importantly, the criteria were originally designed for research purposes to help distinguish different types of vasculitis; yet, they are of no use for making the diagnosis in individual patients [32].

This is at least partially attributable to the fact that frequent symptoms of giant cell arteritis, such as jaw claudication, diplopia, neck pain, and elevated C-reactive protein, were not included in the criteria. In contrast, included criteria, such as headache and scalp tenderness, can be attributable to various other diseases. A normal erythrocyte sedimentation rate does not rule out giant cell arteritis, as has been found in up to 30% of patients with biopsy-proven giant cell arteritis [33,34]. Approximately 40% of the patients with giant cell arteritis present with nonspecific symptomatology that does not apply to any set of criteria. Especially in older patients, systemic giant cell arteritis symptoms like fever, anorexia, weight loss, and malaise may focus the diagnostic workup toward a suspected malignancy [35].

Frequent clinical features of Takayasu's arteritis, such as fever, postural dizziness, arthralgias, weight loss, headache, hypertension, elevated erythrocyte sedimentation rate, and anemia, were not included in the classification criteria of the American College of Rheumatology. Conversely, angiographic findings as well as different blood pressure in each arm are part of the diagnostic criteria; however, false-negative angiograms are frequently found in early vasculitis [36,37], and patients with Takayasu's arteritis restricted to the abdominal aorta or its branches or to the pulmonary artery do not have different blood pressure in each arm.

The wide clinical spectrum and diagnostic limitations frequently cause a delay in diagnosis and subsequent treatment of giant cell arteritis and Takayasu's arteritis. The use of [^{18}F]FDG-PET can possibly increase the diagnostic certainty and speed up the detection of disease activity.

[^{18}F]fluorodeoxyglucose PET

[^{18}F]FDG-PET is an operator-independent noninvasive imaging modality based on the regional distribution of [^{18}F]FDG. Deoxyglucose can be labeled with the positron-emitting radionuclide ^{18}fluor and is administered intravenously to patients after fasting. [^{18}F]FDG initially distributes in proportion to the perfusion of the organs, whereby it follows the same uptake metabolic route as glucose. Although [^{18}F]FDG is phosphorylated to [^{18}F]FDG-6-phosphate, it is not further metabolized. By this mechanism and also because of its low membrane permeability, it becomes trapped and is accumulated within the cells. The emitted positron can be detected by a scanner, and a bright signal in the [^{18}F]FDG-PET scan reflects increased glucose metabolism.

Many malignancies have heightened glucose metabolism, and for several years, this property has allowed functional examination with [^{18}F]FDG-PET, especially for staging and follow-up in various types of cancers [1]. Activated inflammatory cells have also been shown to overexpress glucose transporters and accumulate increased amounts of glucose and structurally related substances, such as [^{18}F]FDG [38,39], which provides an important rationale for the use of [^{18}F]FDG-PET in vasculitis.

[^{18}F]fluorodeoxyglucose PET scanning protocols for large vessel vasculitis

The American Association of Nuclear Medicine and the European Association of Nuclear Medicine have established procedure guidelines for tumor imaging with [^{18}F]FDG-PET [40,41]. The guidelines of the American Association of Nuclear Medicine from 1998 recommend fasting for at least 4 hours before the scan. Low blood glucose levels are recommended, the injected [^{18}F]FDG activity should be 350 to 750 MBq, and the acquisition should be started 30 to 40 minutes after injection. In contrast, the guidelines of the European Association of Nuclear Medicine from 2003 advocate fasting for at least 6 hours before the scan. The blood glucose level should not exceed 130 mg/dL, the injected [^{18}F]FDG activity should be 6 MBq/kg, and acquisition should be started 60 minutes after injection. Guidelines for PET imaging of inflammation, however, are not established by either of these two associations.

Consequently, the present studies [see Table 2] used several different protocols. Prescan fasting intervals of 4 hours [42,43] and 6 hours [44–46] were used. Overnight fasting [47–49] was also utilized. Regarding the applied [^{18}F]FDG dose, body weight-adapted protocols with [^{18}F]FDG at a rate of 5 [48], 6 [49], or 6.5 MBq [45,50] per kilogram of body weight were used, but fixed doses of 296 [51], 370 [47] and 450 [46] MBq were also used. One group routinely administered additional furosemide [44] to accelerate renal [^{18}F]FDG elimination. Most studies on [^{18}F]FDG-PET in large vessel vasculitis did not restrict scanning by maximal glucose levels. Only three studies tolerated maximum serum glucose levels of 100 mg/dL [47,51] and 180 mg/dL [48], respectively. Also, the time interval between [^{18}F]FDG application and image acquisition showed large differences: 45 [48,49], 60 [44,45,47,50,51], and 90 [42,43,46] minutes of [^{18}F]FDG uptake are reported. Generally, dedicated PET scanners with full-ring detectors were used; nevertheless, hybrid cameras have also been successfully employed [47,51,52]. Recently, reports on the use of combined [^{18}F]FDG-PET-CT scanners in large vessel vasculitis have become available [49,53,54].

This summary indicates the present lack of standardization; however, it also demonstrates that [^{18}F]FDG-PET can stably image large vessel vasculitis under a variety of protocols.

[^{18}F]fluorodeoxyglucose PET and atherosclerosis

Not only vasculitic vessels but atherosclerotic plaques have been shown to accumulate glucose analogues [Fig. 1] [55]. As a result, modest large vessel [^{18}F]FDG accumulation at the level of the major vessels occurs in approximately 50% of all PET scans, with increased prevalence in older people [56,57]. This vascular uptake might be explained by smooth muscle metabolism in the media, subendothelial smooth muscle proliferation from senescence, and the presence of macrophages within the atherosclerotic plaque. Thus, vascular uptake found in the [^{18}F]FDG-PET scan is not specific for vasculitis.

Nonetheless, atherosclerotic lesions can be differentiated from vasculitic lesions by taking into account the vascular distribution, the [^{18}F]FDG uptake pattern, and the intensity of [^{18}F]FDG accumulation. For example, the internal carotid artery demonstrates atherosclerotic changes more frequently, whereas the external carotid artery more often reveals inflammatory changes. The uptake pattern of atherosclerotic mediastinal great vessels sometimes can be identified as ring-shaped

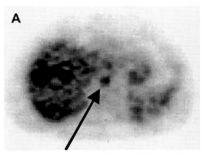
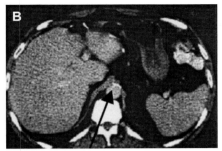

Fig. 1. Axial [18F]FDG-PET images through the abdomen (*A*) show intense FDG activity distributed in the abdominal aorta, whereas the corresponding nonenhanced CT images through the same region (*B*) show the calcified atherosclerotic plaques of the aorta. (*From* Yun M, Yeh D, Araujo LI, et al. F-18 FDG uptake in the large arteries: a new observation. Clin Nucl Med 2001;26(4):314–9; with permission.)

structures. Conversely, the uptake pattern in the arteries of the abdomen and lower extremities is often linear and continuous [56]. Most discriminatingly, atherosclerotic lesions rarely demonstrate intense uptake of FDG [47,48].

Accordingly, to differentiate vasculitis from atherosclerosis, visual scoring of vascular [18F]FDG uptake compared with [18F]FDG accumulation in the liver has been established. Accordingly, 3 grades of large vessel [18F]FDG uptake are differentiated [Fig. 2]: grade I, uptake present but lower than liver uptake; grade II, similar to liver uptake; and grade III, uptake higher than liver uptake. This scale was proposed by Meller and colleagues [47] and was subsequently validated to represent the severity of inflammation [48].

So far, this score has been used in two reference patient populations without clinical symptoms or laboratory signs of large vessel inflammation to determine the uptake in nonvasculitic vessels [47,48]. Thereby, grade I vessel uptake was frequently found in the thoracic part of the aorta, which was most likely attributable to atherosclerosis. Accordingly, only grade II or III [18F]FDG uptake in the thoracic aorta and any visible uptake in other segments should routinely be judged as active large vessel inflammation. In this manner, most lesions can be ruled out as being caused by atherosclerosis. Conversely, computed quantification of [18F]FDG uptake by standard uptake value (SUV) has not been shown to be useful in discriminating atherosclerosis from vasculitis to date.

[18F]fluorodeoxyglucose PET for diagnosing giant cell arteritis

Today, the diagnosis of giant cell arteritis is mainly based on clinical evaluation, laboratory results, and temporal biopsy. In addition, no imaging modality has been included in the American College of Rheumatology diagnostic criteria for giant cell arteritis [see Table 1]. Nevertheless, [18F]FDG-PET has indicated its usefulness in a number of studies with better evidence as compared with Takayasu's arteritis because of the higher frequency of the disease. Currently, the reports on nine studies including 118 patients are available on use of [18F]FDG-PET in giant cell arteritis [see Table 2].

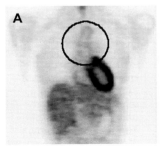
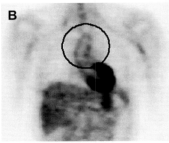
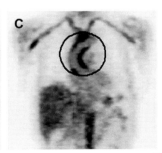

Fig. 2. The visual arteritis score as proposed by Meller and colleagues [47]. The severity of large vessel [18F]FDG uptake is visually graded: grade 1, uptake present but lower than liver uptake (*A*); grade 2, similar to liver uptake (*B*); and grade 3, uptake higher than liver uptake (*C*). (*From* Walter MA, Melzer RA, Schindler C, et al. The value of [18F]FDG-PET in the diagnosis of large-vessel vasculitis and the assessment of activity and extent of disease. Eur J Nucl Med Mol Imaging 2005;32(6):676; with permission.)

The common uptake pattern found in great vessels affected by giant cell arteritis was linear and continuous, and the predominant uptake was grade II. Overall, thoracic vessels were most frequently affected, followed by abdominal vessels [47,48]. The ability to detect large vessel inflammation differed considerably in the available publications. In studies using patient populations with polymyalgia rheumatica and giant cell arteritis, patient sensitivities between 56% and 100% were reported [44,45,50,52], with a specificity between 77% and 98% [50]. These differences can partially be explained by the inclusion of patients with dissimilar activity of the disease. Accordingly, a recent study could confirm that high sensitivities are achieved, especially in the state of active inflammation [Fig. 3]. Thereby, the C-reactive protein has been shown to be a better predictor for the sensitivity of [18F]FDG-PET in giant cell arteritis than the erythrocyte sedimentation rate [48].

Comparative studies using [18F]FDG-PET and MRI revealed comparable sensitivities of the two methods, but [18F]FDG-PET has been shown to identify significantly more affected vascular regions [47,52]. These results reflect the advantage of metabolic imaging, because metabolic changes normally precede morphologic changes in giant cell arteritis. Moreover, [18F]FDG-PET might also allow new insights into the pathologic findings of giant cell arteritis and polymyalgia rheumatica. A study in patients with polymyalgia rheumatica demonstrated inflammation of the aorta or its major branches in 92% of patients. The tracer uptake was strongly correlated to the erythrocyte sedimentation rate and the C-reactive protein. These data indicate that polymyalgia rheumatica is frequently accompanied by subclinical vasculitis [46].

Moreover, [18F]FDG-PET offers the possibility of whole-body screening in one procedure. Thus, it might become helpful in the follow-up of patients with giant cell arteritis. [18F]FDG-PET results have shown good correlation with the clinical course, which was also confirmed by computed quantification of the vascular [18F]FDG accumulation [46]. Compared with the MRI results, the follow-up results of [18F]FDG-PET correlate significantly better with clinical improvement [47], because [18F]FDG-PET is able to monitor changes in metabolic activity directly.

The value of [18F]FDG-PET for diagnosing temporal arteritis has recently been investigated in a study comprising 22 patients [45]. Of these patients, 17 had involvement of the temporal arteries; however, no such involvement was detected by [18F]FDG-PET. This limitation of [18F]FDG-PET is mainly attributable to the high [18F]FDG uptake in the brain and the small diameter of the temporal arteries. Thus, direct evaluation of the temporal arteries does not seem to be feasible with current whole-body PET techniques.

[18F]fluorodeoxyglucose PET for diagnosing Takayasu's arteritis

In contrast to giant cell arteritis, the initial diagnosis of Takayasu's arteritis is partly based on morphologic imaging. The results of angiography are also integrated in the diagnostic criteria of the American College of Rheumatology [see Table 2]. Angiographic alterations usually occur in the late phase of Takayasu's arteritis, however, and metabolic imaging with [18F]FDG-PET facilitates detection of metabolic changes during the early phase. To date, the data on the use of [18F]FDG-PET in Takayasu's

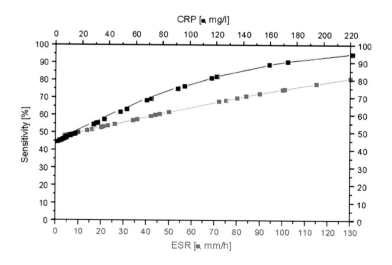

Fig. 3. Sensitivity of large vessel vasculitis. [18F]FDG-PET uptake as a function of the C-reactive protein (CRP) and erythrocyte sedimentation rate (ESR) levels, respectively. High sensitivity for detection of large vessel vasculitis is reached at high CRP and ESR levels. (*From* Walter MA, Melzer RA, Schindler C, et al. The value of [18F]FDG-PET in the diagnosis of large-vessel vasculitis and the assessment of activity and extent of disease. Eur J Nucl Med Mol Imaging 2005;32(6):677; with permission.)

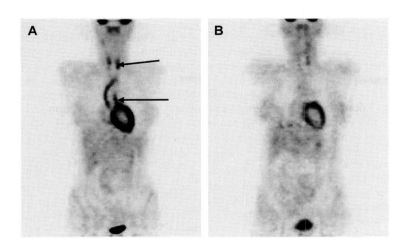

Fig. 4. (*A*) [^{18}F]FDG-PET scan of a patient with Takayasu's arteritis, with markedly abnormal uptake of [^{18}F]FDG in the aortic arch and carotid arteries (*arrows*). (*B*) [^{18}F]FDG-PET scan of the same patient in clinical remission after treatment with prednisone and intravenous cyclophosphamide. (*From* Andrews J, Al-Nahhas A, Pennell DJ, et al. Non-invasive imaging in the diagnosis and management of Takayasu's arteritis. Ann Rheum Dis 2004; 63(8):998; with permission.)

arteritis are poor compared with the data on [^{18}F]FDG-PET in giant cell arteritis because of the rarity of the disease. Only seven studies including a total of 51 patients have been reported on to date.

The common [^{18}F]FDG uptake pattern in the early phase of Takayasu's arteritis is linear and continuous [Fig. 4A], whereas in the late phase, it can become patchy rather than continuous but still in a linear distribution [43]. Based on the present data, the diagnostic value of [^{18}F]FDG-PET seems to be consistently high in Takayasu's arteritis. Two studies reported sensitivities of 83% and 100%

[42,51], whereas another report found a sensitivity of 92%, with a specificity of 100% and a diagnostic accuracy of 94% [43]. These sensitivities are comparable to those of MRI; however, metabolic imaging using [^{18}F]FDG-PET in Takayasu's arteritis has been shown to identify more affected vascular regions than morphologic imaging with MRI [51]. Nevertheless, it has to be mentioned that [^{18}F]FDG-PET does not provide any information about changes in the wall structure or luminal blood flow.

Similar to the situation in giant cell arteritis, there is a clear correlation between the activity of large

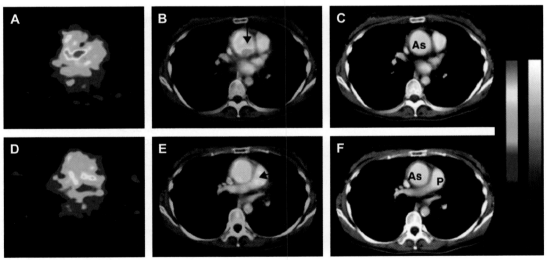

Fig. 5. [^{18}F]FDG-PET scan coregistered with enhanced CT scan of a patient with active Takayasu's arteritis revealed that [^{18}F]FDG accumulations were localized in the vascular wall of the ascending aortic and pulmonary artery. (*A, D*) Axial images of the [^{18}F]FDG-PET with [^{18}F]FDG accumulation in the mediastinum. Coregistered PET scan with enhanced CT images. The arrows indicate [^{18}F]FDG accumulation in the ascending aorta (*B*) and pulmonary arteries (*E*). (*C, F*) Enhanced reconstituted CT images of the same level as A and D. The ascending aorta was enlarged, causing aortic regurgitation. As, ascending aorta; P, pulmonary artery. (*From* Kobayashi Y, Ishii K, Oda K, et al. Aortic wall inflammation due to Takayasu arteritis imaged with 18F-FDG PET coregistered with enhanced CT. J Nucl Med 2005;46(6):919; with permission.)

vessel inflammation and the ability of [^{18}F]FDG-PET to detect inflammatory vessels. In a recent study, [^{18}F]FDG-PET-positive patients showed significantly higher erythrocyte sedimentation rates and C-reactive protein levels as compared with [^{18}F]FDG-PET-negative patients, with the C-reactive protein as a superior marker [43].

A follow-up in Takayasu's arteritis only based on clinical symptoms has been shown to be rather limited. In a previous report, biopsy demonstrated active inflammation in 44% of patients thought to be in clinical remission [58]. Conversely, [^{18}F]FDG-PET is able to detect more sites than just those that were clinically active [43]. Because of its high sensitivity and the good correlation with outcome, [^{18}F]FDG-PET is a promising candidate to be used regularly in the follow-up of Takayasu's arteritis [see Fig. 4] [42,43,48].

[^{18}F]fluorodeoxyglucose PET CT in large vessel vasculitis

The combination of [^{18}F]FDG-PET scanners with CT scanners is becoming increasingly important in the management of oncologic patients [59–61]. The combination of both techniques allows the integration of morphologic and metabolic information for detection, staging, and therapy control. The rapidly increasing availability of [^{18}F]FDG-PET-CT scanners is also introducing new opportunities for their application in rheumatology. The use of combined [^{18}F]FDG-PET-CT scanners should allow the investigation of the morphology and metabolic activity of affected vessels. Moreover, the localization of affected segments should be significantly improved. Two case reports have already indicated the value of [^{18}F]FDG-PET-CT scanners in large vessel vasculitis [52,53], and one clinical trial has investigated the value of the combination of both modalities in 14 patients [49]. The coregistered CT scan was most useful for the anatomic identification of vascular [^{18}F]FDG uptake, especially in the case of rather moderate [^{18}F]FDG accumulation. Furthermore, the anatomic identification of mediastinal [^{18}F]FDG uptake, particularly in the pulmonary arteries, was significantly improved [Fig. 5]. The evaluation of [^{18}F]FDG-PET-CT scanners in large vessel vasculitis is ongoing; however, the first results are quite promising.

Summary

In conclusion, whole-body imaging with [^{18}F]FDG-PET is highly effective in assessing the activity and extent of giant cell arteritis and Takayasu's arteritis, respectively:

Metabolic imaging using [^{18}F]FDG-PET has been shown to identify more affected vascular regions than morphologic imaging with MRI in both diseases.

The visual grading of vascular [^{18}F]FDG uptake helps to discriminate arteritis from atherosclerosis and therefore provides high specificity.

High sensitivity is attained by scanning during the active inflammatory phase.

Thus, [^{18}F]FDG-PET has the potential to develop into a valuable tool in the diagnostic workup of giant cell arteritis and Takayasu's arteritis, respectively, and might become a first-line investigation technique. Consensus regarding the most favorable imaging procedure as well as further clinical evidence is urgently needed, however.

Acknowledgments

The author is grateful to Ralf Melzer, Helmut Rasch, and Allan Tyndall for their most helpful comments on the article.

References

[1] Rohren EM, Turkington TG, Coleman RE. Clinical applications of PET in oncology. Radiology 2004;231(2):305–32.

[2] Turlakow A, Yeung HW, Pui J, et al. Fludeoxyglucose positron emission tomography in the diagnosis of giant cell arteritis. Arch Intern Med 2001;161(7):1003–7.

[3] Blockmans D, Van Moer E, Dehem J, et al. Positron emission tomography can reveal abdominal periaortitis. Clin Nucl Med 2002;27(3):211–2.

[4] Wenger M, Gasser R, Donnemiller E, et al. Images in cardiovascular medicine. Generalized large vessel arteritis visualized by 18 fluorodeoxyglucose-positron emission tomography. Circulation 2003;107(6):923.

[5] Brodmann M, Lipp RW, Aigner R, et al. Positron emission tomography reveals extended thoracic and abdominal peri-aortitis. Vasc Med 2003;8(2):127–8.

[6] Wiest R, Gluck T, Schonberger J, et al. Clinical image: occult large vessel vasculitis diagnosed by PET imaging. Rheumatol Int 2001;20(6):250.

[7] De Winter F, Petrovic M, Van de Wiele C, et al. Imaging of giant cell arteritis: evidence of splenic involvement using FDG positron emission tomography. Clin Nucl Med 2000;25(8):633–4.

[8] Hara M, Goodman PC, Leder RA. FDG-PET finding in early-phase Takayasu arteritis. J Comput Assist Tomogr 1999;23(1):16–8.

[9] Malik IS, Harare O, Al-Nahhas A, et al. Takayasu's arteritis: management of left main stem stenosis. Heart 2003;89(3):e9.

[10] Walter MA, Melzer RA, Graf M, et al. [18F]FDG-PET of giant-cell aortitis. Rheumatology (Oxford) 2005;44(5):690–1.

[11] Hutchinson J. On a peculiar form of thrombotic arteritis of the aged which is sometimes productive or gangrene. Arch Surg 1890;1:323–9.

[12] Klein RG, Hunder GG, Stanson AW, et al. Large artery involvement in giant cell (temporal) arteritis. Ann Intern Med 1975;83(6):806–12.

[13] Salvarani C, Gabriel SE, O'Fallon WM, et al. The incidence of giant cell arteritis in Olmsted County, Minnesota: apparent fluctuations in a cyclic pattern. Ann Intern Med 1995;123(3):192–4.

[14] Franzen P, Sutinen S, von Knorring J. Giant cell arteritis and polymyalgia rheumatica in a region of Finland: an epidemiologic, clinical and pathologic study, 1984–1988. J Rheumatol 1992; 19(2):273–6.

[15] Gonzalez-Gay MA, Alonso MD, Aguero JJ, et al. Giant cell arteritis in Mediterranean countries: comment on the article by Salvarani et al. Arthritis Rheum 1992;35(10):1249–50.

[16] Ostberg G. An arteritis with special reference to polymyalgia arteritica. Acta Pathol Microbiol Scand [A] 1973;237(Suppl 237):1–59.

[17] Lie JT. Illustrated histopathologic classification criteria for selected vasculitis syndromes. American College of Rheumatology Subcommittee on Classification of Vasculitis. Arthritis Rheum 1990;33(8):1074–87.

[18] Weyand CM. The Dunlop-Dottridge Lecture: the pathogenesis of giant cell arteritis. J Rheumatol 2000;27(2):517–22.

[19] Salvarani C, Macchioni PL, Tartoni PL, et al. Polymyalgia rheumatica and giant cell arteritis: a 5-year epidemiologic and clinical study in Reggio Emilia, Italy. Clin Exp Rheumatol 1987; 5(3):205–15.

[20] Huston KA, Hunder GG. Giant cell (cranial) arteritis: a clinical review. Am Heart J 1980; 100(1):99–105.

[21] Calamia KT, Hunder GG. Giant cell arteritis (temporal arteritis) presenting as fever of undetermined origin. Arthritis Rheum 1981;24(11): 1414–8.

[22] Takayasu M. Case with unusual changes of the central vessels in the retina. Acta Soc Ophthal Jpn 1908;12:554–5.

[23] Waern AU, Andersson P, Hemmingsson A. Takayasu's arteritis: a hospital-region based study on occurrence, treatment and prognosis. Angiology 1983;34(5):311–20.

[24] Hall S, Barr W, Lie JT, et al. Takayasu arteritis. A study of 32 North American patients. Medicine (Baltimore) 1985;64(2):89–99.

[25] el-Reshaid K, Varro J, al-Duwairi Q, et al. Takayasu's arteritis in Kuwait. J Trop Med Hyg 1995; 98(5):299–305.

[26] Lande A. Abdominal Takayasu's aortitis, the middle aortic syndrome and atherosclerosis. A critical review. Int Angiol 1998;17(1):1–9.

[27] Nasu T. Pathology of pulseless disease. A systematic study and critical review of twenty-one autopsy cases reported in Japan. Angiology 1963; 14:225–42.

[28] Matsunaga N, Hayashi K, Sakamoto I, et al. Takayasu arteritis: protean radiologic manifestations and diagnosis. Radiographics 1997;17(3): 579–94.

[29] Moriwaki R, Noda M, Yajima M, et al. Clinical manifestations of Takayasu arteritis in India and Japan: new classification of angiographic findings. Angiology 1997;48(5):369–79.

[30] Hunder GG, Bloch DA, Michel BA, et al. The American College of Rheumatology 1990 criteria for the classification of giant cell arteritis. Arthritis Rheum 1990;33(8):1122–8.

[31] Arend WP, Michel BA, Bloch DA, et al. The American College of Rheumatology 1990 criteria for the classification of Takayasu arteritis. Arthritis Rheum 1990;33(8):1129–34.

[32] Rao JK, Allen NB, Pincus T. Limitations of the 1990 American College of Rheumatology classification criteria in the diagnosis of vasculitis. Ann Intern Med 1998;129(5):345–52.

[33] Salvarani C, Hunder GG. Giant cell arteritis with low erythrocyte sedimentation rate: frequency of occurrence in a population-based study. Arthritis Rheum 2001;45(2):140–5.

[34] Hayreh SS, Zimmerman B. Management of giant cell arteritis. Our 27-year clinical study: new light on old controversies. Ophthalmologica 2003; 217(4):239–59.

[35] Gonzalez-Gay MA, Garcia-Porrua C, Salvarani C, et al. The spectrum of conditions mimicking polymyalgia rheumatica in Northwestern Spain. J Rheumatol 2000;27(9):2179–84.

[36] Lambert M, Hachulla E, Hatron PY, et al. [Takayasu's arteritis: vascular investigations and therapeutic management. Experience with 16 patients]. Rev Med Interne 1998;19(12):878–84 [in French].

[37] Lambert M, Hatron PY, Hachulla E, et al. Takayasu's arteritis diagnosed at the early systemic phase: diagnosis with noninvasive investigation despite normal findings on angiography. J Rheumatol 1998;25(2):376–7.

[38] Ishimori T, Saga T, Mamede M, et al. Increased (18)F-FDG uptake in a model of inflammation: concanavalin A-mediated lymphocyte activation. J Nucl Med 2002;43(5):658–63.

[39] Jones HA, Cadwallader KA, White JF, et al. Dissociation between respiratory burst activity and deoxyglucose uptake in human neutrophil granulocytes: implications for interpretation of (18)F-FDG PET images. J Nucl Med 2002; 43(5):652–7.

[40] Schelbert HR, Hoh CK, Royal HD, et al. Procedure guideline for tumor imaging using fluorine-18-FDG. Society of Nuclear Medicine. J Nucl Med 1998;39(7):1302–5.

[41] Bombardieri E, Aktolun C, Baum RP, et al. FDG-PET: procedure guidelines for tumour imaging. Eur J Nucl Med Mol Imaging 2003;30(12): BP115–24.

[42] Andrews J, Al-Nahhas A, Pennell DJ, et al. Noninvasive imaging in the diagnosis and

management of Takayasu's arteritis. Ann Rheum Dis 2004;63(8):995–1000.

[43] Webb M, Chambers A, Al-Nahhas A, et al. The role of 18F-FDG PET in characterising disease activity in Takayasu arteritis. Eur J Nucl Med Mol Imaging 2004;31(5):627–34.

[44] Bleeker-Rovers CP, Bredie SJ, van der Meer JW, et al. F-18-fluorodeoxyglucose positron emission tomography in diagnosis and follow-up of patients with different types of vasculitis. Neth J Med 2003;61(10):323–9.

[45] Brodmann M, Lipp RW, Passath A, et al. The role of 2-18F-fluoro-2-deoxy-D-glucose positron emission tomography in the diagnosis of giant cell arteritis of the temporal arteries. Rheumatology (Oxford) 2004;43(2):241–2.

[46] Moosig F, Czech N, Mehl C, et al. Correlation between 18-fluorodeoxyglucose accumulation in large vessels and serological markers of inflammation in polymyalgia rheumatica: a quantitative PET study. Ann Rheum Dis 2004;63(7):870–3.

[47] Meller J, Strutz F, Siefker U, et al. Early diagnosis and follow-up of aortitis with [(18)F]FDG PET and MRI. Eur J Nucl Med Mol Imaging 2003;30(5):730–6.

[48] Walter MA, Melzer RA, Schindler C, et al. The value of [18F]FDG-PET in the diagnosis of large-vessel vasculitis and the assessment of activity and extent of disease. Eur J Nucl Med Mol Imaging 2005;32(6):674–81.

[49] Kobayashi Y, Ishii K, Oda K, et al. Aortic wall inflammation due to Takayasu arteritis imaged with 18F-FDG PET coregistered with enhanced CT. J Nucl Med 2005;46(6):917–22.

[50] Blockmans D, Stroobants S, Maes A, et al. Positron emission tomography in giant cell arteritis and polymyalgia rheumatica: evidence for inflammation of the aortic arch. Am J Med 2000;108(3):246–9.

[51] Meller J, Grabbe E, Becker W, et al. Value of F-18 FDG hybrid camera PET and MRI in early Takayasu aortitis. Eur Radiol 2003;13(2):400–5.

[52] Scheel AK, Meller J, Vosshenrich R, et al. Diagnosis and follow up of aortitis in the elderly. Ann Rheum Dis 2004;63(11):1507–10.

[53] Kroger K, Antoch G, Goyen M, et al. Positron emission tomography/computed tomography improves diagnostics of inflammatory arteritis. Heart Vessels 2005;20(4):179–83.

[54] Antoch G, Freudenberg LS, Debatin JF, et al. Images in vascular medicine. Diagnosis of giant cell arteritis with PET/CT. Vasc Med 2003;8(4):281–2.

[55] Rudd JH, Warburton EA, Fryer TD, et al. Imaging atherosclerotic plaque inflammation with [18F]-fluorodeoxyglucose positron emission tomography. Circulation 2002;105(23):2708–11.

[56] Yun M, Yeh D, Araujo LI, et al. F-18 FDG uptake in the large arteries: a new observation. Clin Nucl Med 2001;26(4):314–9.

[57] Yun M, Jang S, Cucchiara A, et al. 18F FDG uptake in the large arteries: a correlation study with the atherogenic risk factors. Semin Nucl Med 2002;32(1):70–6.

[58] Kerr GS, Hallahan CW, Giordano J, et al. Takayasu arteritis. Ann Intern Med 1994;120(11):919–29.

[59] Sachelarie I, Kerr K, Ghesani M, et al. Integrated PET-CT: evidence-based review of oncology indications. Oncology (Williston Park) 2005;19(4):481–90.

[60] Macapinlac HA. FDG PET and PET/CT imaging in lymphoma and melanoma. Cancer J 2004;10(4):262–70.

[61] Frank SJ, Chao KS, Schwartz DL, et al. Technology insight: PET and PET/CT in head and neck tumor staging and radiation therapy planning. Nat Clin Pract Oncol 2005;2(10):526–33.

[62] Blockmans D, Maes A, Stroobants S, et al. New arguments for a vasculitic nature of polymyalgia rheumatica using positron emission tomography. Rheumatology (Oxford) 1999;38(5):444–7.

[63] Blockmans D, Baeyens H, Van Loon R, et al. Periaortitis and aortic dissection due to Wegener's granulomatosis. Clin Rheumatol 2000;19(2):161–4.

[64] Belhocine T, Kaye O, Delanaye P, et al. [Horton's disease and extra-temporal vessel locations: role of 18FDG PET scan. Report of 3 cases and review of the literature]. Rev Med Interne 2002;23(7):584–91 [in French].

[65] Blockmans D, de Ceuninck L, Vanderschueren S, et al. Repetitive ^{18}F-fluorodeoxyglucose positron emission tomography in giant cell arteritis: a prospective study of 35 patients. Arthritis Rheum 2006;55:131–7.

RADIOLOGIC
CLINICS
OF NORTH AMERICA

Radiol Clin N Am 45 (2007) 745–749

Index

Note: Page numbers of article titles are in **boldface** type.

doi:10.1016/S0033-8389(07)00117-0

Moving?

Make sure your subscription moves with you!

To notify us of your new address, find your **Clinics Account Number** (located on your mailing label above your name), and contact customer service at:

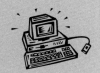

E-mail: elspcs@elsevier.com

800-654-2452 (subscribers in the U.S. & Canada)
407-345-4000 (subscribers outside of the U.S. & Canada)

Fax number: 407-363-9661

Elsevier Periodicals Customer Service
6277 Sea Harbor Drive
Orlando, FL 32887-4800

*To ensure uninterrupted delivery of your subscription, please notify us at least 4 weeks in advance of move.

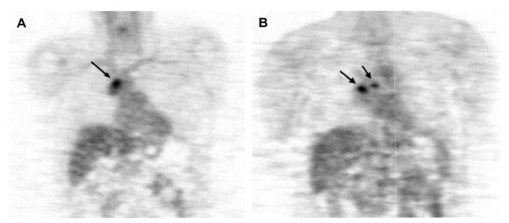

Fig. 3. A 65-year-old man with history of multiple chest wall recurrences of estrogen receptor-positive invasive ductal carcinoma of the right breast. He had undergone multiple chest wall resections, radiation, chemotherapy, and hormonal therapy for these episodes of recurrent disease. Anterior coronal image from FDG-PET (*A*) performed 11 years after original diagnosis of breast cancer shows a focus of uptake in the right anterior chest (*arrow*; SUV = 6.0) consistent with pathologic involvement of an internal mammary node. A more posterior coronal image (*B*) shows two foci of uptake (*arrows*) in the right hilum (SUV = 6.4) and the pretracheal region of the mediastinum (SUV = 5.0).

lesions than bone scintigraphy, except in a subgroup of patients who had osteoblastic metastases. Moreover, the level of FDG uptake in osteolytic lesions was significantly greater compared with osteoblastic lesions, and the prognosis of patients who had osteolytic-predominant disease was significantly worse. A more recent prospective study comparing the sensitivity of FDG-PET with bone single photon emission computed tomography (SPECT) in 15 patients [57] showed a clear superiority of bone SPECT over FDG-PET in sensitivity in detecting skeletal metastases (85% for SPECT versus 17% for FDG), and corroborated the findings of Cook and coworkers regarding the improvement in detection of the subset of osteolytic lesions by FDG-PET. These data clearly show a complementary nature of bone scintigraphy and FDG-PET in the evaluation of skeletal metastases in breast cancer patients [Fig. 4]. These results also suggest that FDG-PET and bone scan should not be considered substitutes for each other for bone metastasis staging in breast cancer. In the author's center, bone scintigraphy remains one of the routine studies in breast cancer metastatic staging, with FDG-PET to help clarify staging in the case of difficult or equivocal conventional staging. Evolving data suggest that [F-18]-fluoride PET may provide similar and likely improved bone metastasis detection in breast cancer and other tumors compared with bone scintigraphy [58,59], and may play a role in breast cancer bone metastasis staging in the future.

Several studies have shown that whole-body FDG-PET is a highly accurate method compared with CI for restaging patients who have previously undergone primary treatment for breast cancer. Results of these studies are summarized in Table 1. One advantage of FDG-PET is that large areas can be surveyed; it is therefore able to evaluate sites of recurrent disease that can be extensive and separated by large anatomic distances. Several investigations have shown the added benefit of FDG-PET to CI in asymptomatic patients who had elevated tumor marker serum levels and negative or equivocal CI [4,7,8]. Although the ability of FDG-PET to successfully detect skeletal metastases compared with bone scintigraphy has been mixed in these series, as previously discussed, FDG-PET has been proven significantly more accurate in the evaluation of nodal disease, and equal or superior to CI for visceral metastases [3,9,50]. In a retrospective study of 61 patients, Vranjesevic and colleagues [60] showed that FDG-PET is significantly more accurate than a combination of CI studies in predicting the outcome (disease-free survival) of patients being re-evaluated after primary treatment of breast cancer. These data support the practice at the author's institution of using FDG-PET as a complement to CI for the evaluation of patients who have suspected recurrent disease.

Impact of F-18 fluorodeoxyglucose-positron emission tomography on patient management

A distinguishing feature of the management of breast cancer is the need for a multidisciplinary

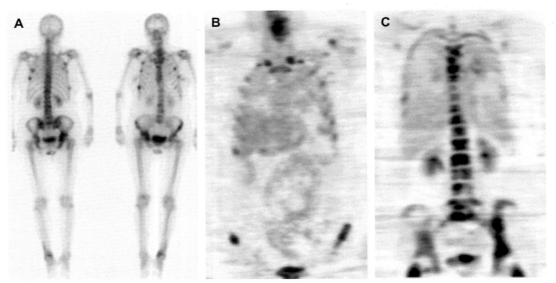

Fig. 4. A 43-year-old woman with bone-dominant metastatic breast cancer. The posterior and anterior projections of bone scan (*A*) show widespread foci of uptake in the axial skeleton and ribs consistent with metastatic disease. Anterior (*B*) and posterior (*C*) coronal images from FDG-PET performed 1 week after the bone scan show much more extensive involvement of the axial skeleton, with a predominant intramedullary uptake pattern in the spine. The pattern of uptake in the ribs is also different compared with the bone scan. The bone scan shows discrete foci in multiple ribs bilaterally that are not as apparent on FDG-PET; these sites represent areas of active cortical bone remodeling from either sclerotic metastases or pathologic fractures. The rib activity in the FDG-PET scan is more diffuse and less discrete, consistent with intramedullary metastases.

approach for optimal local and regional control of the disease. Many strategies and agents offer patients who have advanced breast cancer a therapeutic benefit, including surgery, radiation, chemotherapy, and hormonal therapy. Choosing the most appropriate therapy depends primarily on accurately defining the extent of disease. As of October, 2002, PET has been approved for payment by the Center for Medicare and Medicaid Services in the United States for staging or restaging of patients who have recurrent or metastatic disease, especially when conventional staging studies are equivocal. Despite this approval, there is relatively little insight into which patients who have recurrent or metastatic

Table 1: Studies comparing the ability of whole-body FDG-PET with conventional imaging to detect loco-regional and distant recurrences in patients who have previously undergone primary treatment for breast cancer

Study	Number of patients	Confirmed positive/negative cases	FDG-PET Sensitivity (TP/TP + FN)[a]	FDG-PET Specificity (TN/TN + FP)[a]
Bender et al [2]	75	60/15	95% (41/43)	96% (213/221)
Moon et al [3]	57	29/28	93% (27/29)	79% (22/28)
Lonneux et al [4]	39[b]	33/6	94% (31/33)	50% (3/6)
Kim et al [5]	27	17/10	94% (16/17)	80% (8/10)
Lin et al [6]	36	11/25	85% (23/27)	96% (85/89)
Liu et al [7]	30[b]	28/2	89% (25/28)	50% (1/2)
Suarez et al [8]	38[b]	26/12	92% (24/26)	75% (9/12)
Gallowitsch et al [9]	62	34/28	97% (33/34)	82% (23/28)
Siggelkow et al [10]	57	31/26	81% (25/31)	96% (25/26)
Kamel et al [11]	60	43/17	89% (24/27) LRR	84% (16/19) LRR
			100% (26/26) DM	97% (30/31) DM

Abbreviations: DM, distant metastases; FN, false negative; FP, false positive; LRR, loco-regional recurrence; TN, true negative; TP, true positive.
[a] Values calculated on patient analysis except in [2] and [6], in which values are calculated on lesion analysis.
[b] Patients were mostly or all asymptomatic with elevated tumor markers.